3.50

Suspect

Dr Sam Rosen

# The Autobiography
# of Dr. Samuel Rosen

# The Autobiography

# of Dr. Samuel Rosen

ALFRED A. KNOPF · NEW YORK · 1973

THIS IS A BORZOI BOOK
PUBLISHED BY ALFRED A. KNOPF, INC.

Library of Congress Cataloging in Publication Data

Rosen, Samuel, (date)
    The autobiography of Dr. Samuel Rosen.

    1.  Rosen, Samuel, 1897–    2.  Otolaryngologists—Correspondence,
reminiscences, etc.
RF38.R67A3        617.8'00924 [B]        72-11041
ISBN 0-394-44343-8

Manufactured in the United States of America
First Edition

**For Helen**

*None so deaf as those who will not hear.*

—ENGLISH PROVERB

- - - - - - - - - - - - - - - - - - - - - - - - - - - - - - - - - - - - - - - - - - - - - - - - - - - - - - - - - - - - - - - - - - - - - - -

*A man may see how this world goes with no eyes. Look with thine ears: see how yon justice rails upon yon simple thief. Hark, in thine ear: change place; and handy-dandy, which is the justice, which is the thief?*

—KING LEAR, ACT IV: SCENE 6

# Contents

x · **Contents**

# Illustrations

# Acknowledgments

I should like to express here my grateful appreciation to the many physicians, nurses, audiologists, and laymen, and the many organizations and individuals whose encouragement and assistance have made possible a rewarding career in medicine and medical research. It is clearly impossible to name them all. They live in many lands and come from all walks of life. If, in expressing my appreciation to the few who are mentioned below, I have overlooked any who ought to have been specially recognized, I offer my apologies.

Those whom I wish particularly to thank are:

The late George and Ella Rosen, the late Maurice Rosen, and Harry, Fanny, and Jacob Rosen, whose joint efforts provided a "Rosen scholarship fund" that enabled me to earn my M.D. The late Isadore and Laura Friesner, whose guidance and example sustained me early in my career. The late Henry A. Wallace, who honored me with intellectual and scientific companionship as well as devoted friendship. All my patients, whose confidence in my skill was matched by their willingness to undergo sometimes new and only partially proven techniques, thereby enabling me to improve methods of ear surgery for the benefit of others. George Baehr, whose timely intervention made it possible for me to develop stapes surgery much more rapidly than would have been the case had I been unable to conduct hundreds of experimental operations on cadavers. All of those silent ones whose gift to the living can never be adequately acknowledged. Benjamin Volk and Stewart Nash, who saw to it that I received a hearing before juries of my scientific peers. The late William Chapman White, Roland Berg, and Albert Rosenfeld, among other science writers, who presented my work accurately to the lay public at the proper time. The African Medical and Research Foundation and the Samuel Rubin Foundation, both of which generously aided my studies in remote parts of the world. Belle Sien and Marvel Cooke, who unfailingly carried out often tedious duties in running my office and deciphering a physician's traditionally illegible hand. Albert G. and Judith V. Ruben, John F. Rosen, and Robert and Margaret Stieefel, who encouraged me in my work and in undertaking this book. Martha Gillmor, who provided valuable editorial advice. Linda J. Paton, who typed the manuscript accurately and swiftly. Angus Cameron, who persistently declined to take No for an answer and whose reward—for what it is worth— is this volume. Helen v. Rosen, who has served the world over as audiologist, operating room assistant, logistics expert, and intellectual and emotional companion.

The conversations reported in quotation marks in this book are, of course, not the exact words of the speakers. No one could possibly recall precisely what was said after many years have passed. I have not attempted to do so, but I have tried to make the quoted words as close a paraphrase of what actually transpired as a scrupulous effort to be accurate permits.

Finally, I want particularly to acknowledge the collaborative role of Daniel S. Gillmor, whose expertise as a science writer and editorial assistant have become very much a part of this book.

S.R.

*New York, 1973*

# The Autobiography
# of Dr. Samuel Rosen

# Of Unexpected Journeys

Life is a journey that no one elects to take. It is thrust upon us, and so are its events, few of which turn out to be what we had expected. This book, for example, is not the book I thought it would be when I first thought of writing it, no more than my life has been what I expected it to be. Every man's life, it seems to me, is a series of accidents. If a young woman had not been assigned to me as a patient when I was a resident, my whole life would have been utterly different. A discussion in a hospital cafeteria led to a line of thought which led, in turn, to a preliminary operation whose wholly unexpected outcome abruptly changed my entire career.

We soon learn to discount our fondest dreams for the future, yet even that expectation can turn out to be false. Everyone, for example, who sets out to be a physician secretly hopes that the time will come when he or she is acclaimed as a benefactor of mankind. Then come the years of medical school, the long hours of learning, and later the even longer, more rigorous hours of training. By the time the average doctor has completed the requirements that entitle him to call himself a specialist, he has a very different idea of the price of scientific glory.

Some are not willing to pay it at all. Others by then have decisively concluded that their mission in life is to cure those who can benefit from their knowledge of healing and to give relief from suffering and pain to those for whom medical science as yet has no complete answer. Still others pursue research interests, usually not so much in search of fame as in compulsive pursuit of the answers to mysteries that have caught their curious minds and will not let them go until the riddle is solved and some new secret of nature has been laid bare.

For all of us, I suspect, the first, secret hope lingers, but for most of us it remains just that—a hope, and a forlorn one.

I am one of those lucky ones for whom the hope became a reality. After some thirty years of really quite conventional practice of my specialty—otology, or ear surgery—the unexpected happened to me and to one of my patients in a New York City operating room. The unexpected changed not only my patient's life and my own but also the lives of millions of deaf persons the world over.

I describe the event as something that happened, and so it was. Yet it was not just an accident—nor was subsequent benefit to so many hard of hearing patients the result of mere chance. They were both the product of an attribute common to all doctors, the worst of us and the best. Someone has called it the "therapeutic itch," the insatiable urge to cure. For years people afflicted with partial deafness came to me hoping to be cured by surgery, and for all those years I had to explain to them that only a complicated operation held any hope for even a partial restoration of their hearing.

But since that day in the operating room, I—and my colleagues in otology the world over—can actually cure many of these victims of a certain kind of deafness.

Sometimes an operation that I devised and that others have contributed to can completely or partially restore the hearing of those whose hearing impairment is caused by otosclerosis—a hardening or overgrowth of bone in the middle ear. Sometimes I cannot help them by surgery, because their deafness is the result of damage to the nerve of hearing, located deep within the inner ear, rather than of otosclerosis, which affects the functioning mechanism of the middle ear.

Since I first developed the technique of stapes mobilization in 1952, thousands of patients and doctors have come to me from all over the United States and from many parts of the world. Others could not come, so I have gone to them: to Israel and Egypt; Russia and Spain; India, Jordan, Italy, Hong Kong, Japan, Finland, Cuba, Canada. The list has grown to some forty countries. In each one surgeons come to learn the latest methods of performing this operation. They observe the actual procedure on living patients. Later they ask me questions, listen to my explanations, and then usually we go down to the hospital morgue where they begin the laborious task of acquiring the technique themselves by practicing it on the dead.

I have been doing this for more than fifteen years. Estimating conservatively, I must have performed at least ten thousand stapes mobilizations myself, no two of them presenting exactly the same problem. The doctors to whom I have taught the procedure number in the hundreds and they too have done thousands of operations, while the younger men whom they have taught in turn have restored hearing to thousands more. So you see I am not only the "father" of this surgical procedure; I am its grandfather and great-grandfather.

When I operate in this country, I charge a fee except for those who cannot pay. Everywhere else, I operate and teach without fee, and I travel at my own expense, sometimes aided by funds donated for that purpose by generous patients and friends. And because stapes mobilization requires the use of a specially constructed set of instruments, I take extra sets with me to present to my colleagues abroad.

This has not made me rich, but it has made me enormously proud and happy. I like to think that I am directly or indirectly responsible for restoring to the world of sound literally at least one million human beings.

Even with all this experience, it is still difficult for me truly to comprehend what it is like to be hard of hearing or completely deaf. (The two conditions are not the same, either medically or psychologically.)

My wife Helen and I were fortunate to know Helen Keller, to whom we were introduced by Jo Davidson when he was sculpting his famous portrait of Miss Keller. The two Helens became friends almost instantly. Miss Keller had been blind and deaf from infancy. Her world contained neither light nor sound, but she never ceased her extraordinary effort to maintain contact with the world through the senses left to her.

She delighted in showing off her garden at her home in Connecticut. One day she and Helen Rosen were in the garden, for instance, and Miss Keller, relying entirely on her sense of smell, pointed out the roses, the tulips, the other flowers. She spoke in a harsh, guttural voice, which, of course, she could not hear. At first, the animal-like sound of it added to the strangeness one felt about Miss Keller, but soon one became accustomed to her way of speaking. Then the force of her courage and her indomitable will had their full impact.

All of her awareness of others flowed through her supple hands. She touched you when you met. Her fingers caressed your body, your clothing, your face. When you spoke, she lay her fingertips lightly on your throat or lips. Her touch was delicate, as if aware that privacy was not to be invaded, yet insistent in its demand for contact. You immediately felt that here was a woman whom you could trust.

When my Helen got to know her well, she asked whether

she felt the loss of sight was worse than the loss of hearing. "My dear," Miss Keller said, "you can touch a rose. You can smell it. You do not have to see or hear it to know it. But not to hear a fellow human being's voice is the greatest of deprivations."

She said this with regret, but without perceptible sadness. She had never known what it is to hear, and could only use her powerful intellect to imagine what the sensations of hearing must be like. She had none of the stark realization that the adult who becomes hard of hearing has of what it means to lose contact with the world of sound.

Of his own deafness, for instance, Jonathan Swift wrote bitterly:

*Deaf, giddy, helpless, left alone,*
*To all my friends a burden grown;*
*No more I hear my church's bell*
*Than if it rang out for my knell;*
*At thunder now no more I start*
*Than at the rumbling of a cart;*
*And what's incredible, alack!*
*No more I hear a woman's clack.*

Swift was ruefully reporting what psychologists have also observed: that hearing connects us with the world around us in a way that no other of the five senses does. Even in sleep, auditory sensations continue to reach the brain, maintaining, at least at the unconscious level, an uninterrupted sensory coupling with the environment.

This growing sense of alienation from one's fellow man would be enough to explain why adults who have become hard of hearing are almost always extremely depressed; but, as Dr. D. A. Ramsdell, a clinical psychologist, has pointed out,* the

* In *Hearing and Deafness*, Hallowell Davis, M.D., and S. Richard Silverman, Ph.D., eds. (revised edn.; New York: Holt, Rinehart and Winston, Inc., 1960), pp. 459–73.

depression "is usually more serious than we should expect from the loss of easy two-way communication." He believes that the characteristic personality change which occurs in hard of hearing adults is best explained by noting that hearing occurs simultaneously on three levels: the social level, the signal (or warning) level, and the primitive (or preconscious) level. He describes the primitive level of hearing as a reaction "to the changing background sounds of the world around us *without being aware that we hear them.*" This primitive hearing function enables us to maintain a state of constant readiness to react to the environment, Dr. Ramsdell points out, while at the same time it serves to keep the individual constantly in touch with an ever-changing environment. It follows that the loss of hearing is accompanied by feelings of extreme insecurity about one's place in the surrounding world and of severe depression as a result of the loss of auditory contact with the environment. The world seems to have become lifeless. The deaf person feels deadened inside his soundless world.

The psychoanalysts also attach great importance to hearing in their theory of the development of human personality. The argument essentially goes this way: The eighth cranial nerve supplies the brain with stimuli that come both from the semicircular canals (the organ of equilibrium) and from the inner ear. Study of the evolution of animal species shows that the primitive vestibular organs of, for example, crustaceans, function to provide a static apparatus, an organ that enables the animal to orient itself in space. Man's hearing apparatus is an extension of this primitive organ. He still has an organ of equilibrium and has, in addition, an elaborate hearing mechanism that has special significance for the human being in orienting himself to the world around him.

Specifically, analysts regard the whole auditory mechanism —the outer, middle, and inner ear, and the nerve pathways and their termini in the cortex of the brain—as, in effect, an organ system that permits the infant and the child to develop a psychological equilibrium, a set of moral and ethical values instilled in him through language. The child listens to the sounds of speech. In other words he acquires a language, from which he develops patterns of thought that are common to his culture and a conscience that speaks to him with that well-known "still small voice."

This fascinating idea is reinforced by two other observations, one anatomical, the other psychological. Studies of the structure of the brain show that it is precisely the areas of the cerebral cortex to which the auditory nerve radiates that are the very parts of the brain that differ most in men as compared to apes and other primates. Presumably, these anatomical differences account for man's unique linguistic ability. Psychological observation also reveals another consistent pattern peculiar to man alone: he develops language not only as a means of communication with his fellows but as his own internal mode of communicating with himself—as the pattern of his thoughts. We think largely in words. People who speak several languages find themselves thinking in the language, even though it be a foreign one, that they are currently using most of the time. Finally, the analysts point out, patients who have become psychotic frequently show characteristic symptoms involving their auditory perceptions. They become acutely sensitized to inflection and intonation in the voice of another person and often attribute hostility to what they suppose these phonetic variations imply. In more advanced illnesses, psychotic patients sometimes attribute a deep, secret meaning to what they hear, and even "mishear" what is being said. Ultimately, they reach a point where they develop outright auditory hallucinations in which they are entirely convinced that they hear a warning, admonishing, often derogatory voice speaking to them all the time.

It is beyond the scope of this book and beyond the

competence of an ear surgeon to enlarge on this. But evidently my colleagues in psychological medicine attribute a great deal of importance to what Dr. Otto Isakower once called "the exceptional position of the auditory sphere."* Be that as it may, it is certainly true that hearing and speech are profoundly involved in the processes by which we perceive ourselves in relation to the world around us.

Observation of patients in whom I have been able to restore normal or near-normal hearing by surgery most certainly seems to confirm Dr. Ramsdell's idea of three levels of hearing and the psychological significance of their loss. When hearing returns, the patient is like a prisoner released after many years of confinement.

One of my patients told me a story that illustrates vividly what the experience of restored hearing can mean. I had finished testing her hearing about two weeks after her operation, and we were sitting in my consulting room having a little mutual congratulation session, because the tests showed objectively what she had reported to me: that in her operated ear her hearing was now completely normal.

"Dr. Rosen, did you know there's a click just before the traffic light changes from red to green?" she asked.

"No," I said. "What do you mean 'There's a click'?"

She laughed delightedly: "You're as bad as my husband. You don't really listen to things either!"

Then she told me that she had been driving in New York with her husband. They stopped for a red light, and, a second or two before the light changed, she distinctly heard a click.

"Did you hear that click?" she asked her husband.

Same answer: "No. What click? I didn't hear any click."

At the next red light he listened for the click but he still did not hear it.

* "On the Exceptional Position of the Auditory Sphere," *International Journal of Psycho-Analysis*, Vol. XX, 1939, Parts 3 & 4, pp. 1–9.

"I don't hear any click," he insisted. "You must be imagining it."

"No, I'm sure I hear it," the wife said firmly. "Now next time you really *listen*."

At the third red light the husband listened intently, and sure enough, he heard the click.

"Well, what do you know!" he said. "There *is* a click. I never heard that before in my life, honey. I guess I never really listened for it."

They were both delighted with this silly little episode. Imagine the satisfaction the wife had in being the one to give her husband a novel experience in hearing, the very sense in which she had been so deficient. The triviality of the experience meant absolutely nothing in comparison to the pleasure of communicating.

And in addition there was the confidence she had gained in her new ability to hear. She could say to her husband, "Now you *listen* and you'll hear it." All those years of growing shyness and anxiety she had lived through were banished by the mechanism of a traffic light. Gone in that instant were all those frustrating dialogues:

"What did you say, dear?"

"It wasn't important, never mind."

Patients do not always recount intimate experiences of this kind, and a wise doctor does not ask impertinent questions— "impertinent" either in the sense of impolite or in the sense of not relevant. An essential skill in medical practice is to know when to mind your own business and when to be a gentle but insistent questioner; when to keep out of a patient's private life and when to be a good listener. I have been fortunate in having listened to many moving stories told me by patients whose hearing has been restored.

Some are instructive as well. Many confirm the fact that, although our environment is full of changing patterns of sound, most of us hear them without really listening to them. We are unaware of what we are missing until we really pay attention, like the woman's husband. To a person who is hearing all these sounds for the first time in years, the downright deliciousness of even the most commonplace sounds floods into consciousness: the joy of hearing rain dash against the kitchen window, the sounds of the city at night, of birds at dawn, the squeak of boots in snow, above all, those myriad aural clues that keep telling us that the world around is alive and that we are not alone, and especially that "softest music," the voice of someone we love. "My husband sings in the shower," a patient told me wonderingly. You would have thought she had discovered a new Caruso.

Other patients find their new ability to hear an ironic experience at first. One reported that she had never realized how noisy her refrigerator was. Another said that when she got home from the hospital and turned on the kitchen tap, the noise absolutely terrified her for a moment or two. A journalist who had been hard of hearing for twenty-five years found his own newspaper a source of extreme annoyance. It wasn't the bad news it constantly reported, it was the sound of it when his wife sat at breakfast reading it. "Can't you stop crackling the pages that way?" he snapped. He found it hard to believe that "all that racket" was the natural accompaniment of reading the morning's quota of war, crime, and man's general inhumanity to his fellow man. As he got used to the sound of the paper, he decided that at least it was no worse than the news in it.

Speaking of news, another thing I have noticed about patients whom surgery has relieved of the handicap of severe hearing loss is that they can take personal bad news with much more equanimity than most people. Little troubles, even big troubles, don't get them down to the extent that they depress so-called normal people.

One patient came to my office for a postoperative checkup and announced—with a grin—that she would have to move.

"My goodness," I said. "If I never move again in my life it will be too soon."

"I hate it too," she said, still smiling, "but until after the operation, I didn't realize that my next-door neighbor is a concert pianist. He practices for hours every day and the sound comes right through the walls. You can't get away from it anywhere in my apartment. I'll just have to move."

Other patients give up riding the subway for a time, until they can bear its truly ugly, almost painful din and screech. Others find the noises of air conditioners, trucks, buses, elevators, even typewriters almost intolerable at first. One patient found the sound of a flushing toilet hideously raucous.

"I haven't heard that for twenty years," she said. "I'm not sure you did me such a big favor, Dr. Rosen."

We laughed together at this. We had laughed together before her operation, but this time she could not only see me laugh, she could hear the precise quality of my laughter. She could tell that I appreciated the joke, that I understood completely that she was really enjoying the whole world of sound —everything from Jascha Heifetz to the gurgle and glunk of the plumbing.

# Of a Long, Short Journey

-----------------------------------------------------------------------------

For centuries researchers have investigated how we hear, how we are able to tell one sound from another—a flushing toilet from a masterfully played violin. We still don't know. The path from the known to the unknown begins in a little dark hole in the center of the convoluted ridges of the external ear (see Figure 1). The hole is the opening to a bony canal, lined with skin and wax, that picks up sound waves and amplifies them by reverberation, like the pipe of an organ, until the waves reach the eardrum at the base of the canal. The amplifying property of the canal is the first of several steps by which the ear transforms airborne sound waves into vibrations capable of crossing the barrier between the air-filled external and middle ear and the fluid-filled inner ear.

Just behind the pearly, slightly conical eardrum is a space so small that four or five drops of water would fill it completely. Yet between the inner surface of the drum and the bony wall of the inner ear lie three leverlike bones, suspended

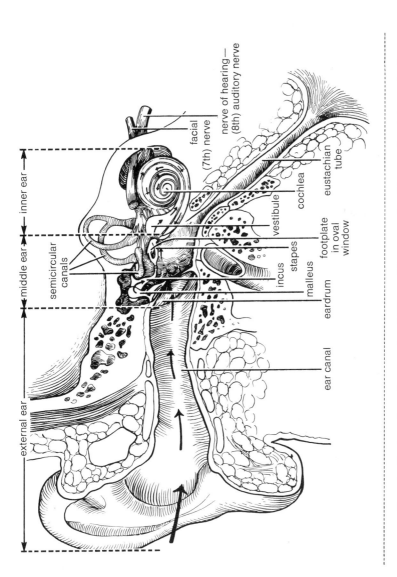

FIGURE 1. *Longitudinal section of external, middle, and inner ear. In this case the right ear is shown. Arrows show the pathway followed by sound entering from the outside.*

external ear

middle ear

inner ear

semicircular canals

nerve of hearing— (8th) auditory nerve

facial (7th) nerve

vestibule

cochlea

eustachian tube

footplate in oval window

stapes

incus

malleus

eardrum

ear canal

and held rigid by eight ligaments and two muscles. And that's not all. Nature, the great improviser, also uses the space as a passageway for two nerves, neither of which apparently has anything to do with auditory functions. They are the facial nerve, injury to which during surgery will cause temporary or permanent paralysis of one side of the patient's face, and the chorda tympani nerve, which serves the sense of taste in a part of the tongue. Behind the middle ear, protected by a wall of the hardest bone in the human body, lies the inner ear, a vaguely snail-shaped organ imbedded in the temporal bone of the skull. Its spiral chamber is divided by a membrane along which hairlike cells detect the motion imparted to the chamber's fluid content by the third of the three middle-ear bones. We know a great deal about the architecture of this inner spiral staircase of the cochlea—and next to nothing about precisely how it functions to convert the vibrations within the chamber into nerve impulses that enable us to distinguish hollow from hearty laughter.

With vibrating tuning forks or using an electronic device and earphones, the ear specialist compares what the patient hears when the sound is presented to the external ear as airborne sound with what he hears when the sound is transmitted directly to the inner ear by setting up vibrations in the skull. (The skull is set to vibrating by touching the base of the humming tuning fork to the mastoid bone just behind the ear, or by applying the fork to the midline of the skull at the forehead.) Broadly speaking, if the patient hears faint sounds equally well by air and bone routes, he is normal. If he hears poorly by air but well by bone conduction, the otologist suspects that the transformer mechanism is at fault: either the external ear canal is blocked, or something has gone wrong in the middle ear. If the patient hears sounds equally well by both routes, but only at much higher than normal volume, the ear specialist suspects that the deafness is due to damage to the delicate structures of the inner ear or to the nerve of hearing itself, both of which are still beyond the reach of surgical or medical help at this stage of otological knowledge.

Before the age of antibiotics, a great deal of damage to the middle-ear mechanism resulted from suppurative infections. If the disease got out of control, it often penetrated the porous mastoid bone behind the ear. From there, invading organisms posed the threat of infecting the covering of the brain, causing meningitis, or of reaching the brain itself and forming a brain abscess. Either complication usually resulted in death.

No wonder, then, that in the pre-antibiotic era we watched our patients and worried over them. Many a night I spent on house calls to such patients, returning home full of anxiety concerning some whose earaches did not respond to my efforts to relieve the pain and pressure of the middle-ear infection. Sometimes it seemed to me that I had just fallen asleep when the phone would ring. A mother was calling. Her child's ear was flaring up again. Would I please come over right away? One night—or rather, early one morning—this happened. I tried to slip out of bed without waking Helen, but she got up and made tea while I dressed. It was just as well that she got up.

"Sit down a minute and drink it before you go," Helen said.

We chatted for a moment or two while I gulped, but my concern about the patient would give me no peace.

"I have to run, honey," I said, as I picked up my bag.

"All right, darling," Helen said good-naturedly, "but don't you think it would be a good idea to put on your pants?"

For years surgeons fought a grim battle against the invader by performing radical operations on the mastoid bone. The idea was to clear out the site of infection so as to permit the patient's natural defenses against disease to overwhelm the now-weakened invading infection. But even when this was a success, the infection often left the middle ear so seriously damaged that impaired hearing was the lasting sequel.

The other leading cause of middle-ear deafness is otosclerosis. This is a disease whose cause is still not understood. All we know is that in some people the bony wall separating the middle and inner ears starts to thicken. If none of the

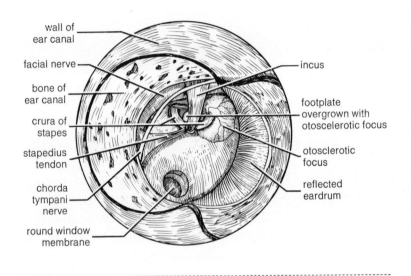

wall of ear canal

facial nerve

bone of ear canal

crura of stapes

stapedius tendon

chorda tympani nerve

round window membrane

incus

footplate overgrown with otoscelerotic focus

otosclerotic focus

reflected eardrum

FIGURE 2. *View of middle ear through operating microscope as seen by stapes surgeon after he has reflected the eardrum. The otosclerotic bony disease for which stapes surgery is ideal is shown at right.*

vital parts of the middle ear become involved, then there are usually no symptoms and the otosclerotic process may never be discovered during the person's lifetime. But if the thickening process encroaches upon the oval window of the vestibule, in which rests the footplate of the tiny stirrup-shaped bone called the stapes, there is trouble (see Figure 2). Gradually, the stapes becomes immobilized. Less and less sound reaches and mobilizes the fluid of the inner ear by the air-conduction route, because the efficiency of the transformer mechanism is gradually being reduced by the encroachment of bone.

The stapes (pronounced "stay-peas") is the last of the three bones whose lever action plays a part in transforming airborne sound. These three bones are linked together by ingeniously balanced joints that carry energy from the vibrating eardrum to the oval window to the inner ear, where the energy is imparted to the fluid within. The minute middle-ear bones are called ossicles and have been named—not very descriptively, except for the stapes—the malleus (hammer), incus (anvil), and stapes (stirrup).

This sound-conduction apparatus—eardrum and ossicles— is a marvel of adaptation to the problem of picking up airborne sound, transforming its energy to overcome the impedance of the inner-ear fluid, and protecting the latter's delicate structures from the damage that would be caused by sudden very loud sounds. The eardrum, for example, is about thirty times the area of the footplate of the stapes, so that the energy gathered by the drum is concentrated in a minute space, so small that a dozen footplates would barely cover the surface of the average adult little fingernail. The stapes, in fact, is the smallest bone in the body. But in addition to the difference in size between drum and footplate, the lever action of the ossicles further transforms the energy transmitted by the drum, changing the vibrations from light, broad movements into short, sharp movements. This lever action resembles the way an automobile jack changes the low-energy, pumping action of its long handle into short, intense energy so powerful it can lift a 4,000-pound car off the ground.

The inner ear has two windows, for otherwise the almost incompressible fluid, called perilymph, could not vibrate in response to the motion of the footplate of the stapes. Both windows have "window panes." The oval window's consists of the stapes footplate, surrounded by an oval ligament, called the annular ligament because it is ring-shaped. The round window is covered by a thin membrane. If the stapes is free to move in its window but all the rest of the middle-ear structures—drum, malleus, and incus—are destroyed, severe loss of hearing results. If the inner ear remains unharmed, the patient can wear a bone-conduction hearing aid so that sounds reach the inner ear directly, instead of via the disrupted air-conduction route. Such damage to the middle-ear mechanism occurs occasionally as a result of accident or illness. And as I have said, it often used to occur as a consequence of infection.

A similar loss of hearing results when otosclerotic overgrowth of the bone freezes the footplate in its window, gradually cutting off transmission of vibration to the inner ear. This doesn't happen all at once. Usually the signs of otosclerosis appear early in adulthood, in the patient's teens or twenties, rarely later than the thirties. The disease may progress rapidly or slowly; it may begin and then fail to progress at all for a long time. It may impede the movement of the footplate but not totally; or it may so completely invade the annular ligament and the footplate that there is absolutely no motion. In other words, it is a very unpredictable disease.

Still, we do know one or two things about it. It never retreats spontaneously; the patient who has otosclerotic deafness at thirty will almost certainly be deafer at forty and will certainly not be able to hear better, unless something is done about it. It also definitely runs in families; the patient with otosclerosis is extremely likely to have a close relative who also has or had the disease. It is much more common among Caucasians than among blacks or Orientals. We used also to think that it was far more common in women than in men, but recent studies indicate that this idea is somewhat exaggerated, although it definitely does occur somewhat more often in women. Furthermore, pregnancy seems to act sometimes as a kind of trigger mechanism that sets the disease in motion.

It would be nice if we could be more specific about otosclerosis, but that is a temptation that we have to resist until we really know more. There is still a lot that we don't know about this form of hearing loss, just as there is almost everything yet to be learned about neurosensory loss. This does not mean that medical scientists don't keep trying to find out. They do. They have been trying for a long time.

# Of Success and Failure

--------------------------------------------------------------------

Success in medicine, as everyone knows, does not come overnight. As a matter of fact, although ear surgeons had long wanted to do something about deafness caused by middle-ear infection, injury, or overgrowth of bone, their most ingenious efforts were frustrated for at least half a century. But doctors are a stubborn lot; at least, some of them are. At about the same time that crude surgical attempts to free the stapes were being roundly condemned, others were thinking of ways to construct some alternate pathway around the frozen stapes and its footplate. If you can't go at it directly, they reasoned, how about indirectly? By the 1900's, carefully performed operations on the mastoid bone were proving that you could not only operate on the ear to relieve the disastrous consequences of infection; you could also invade this critical region of the skull without causing infection—provided you were meticulous in following aseptic surgical techniques.

The way around the blocked oval window was obvious

to some surgeons who knew the anatomy of the inner ear. Right next to the cochlea, and connected to it by a watery passageway termed the vestibule, lie the semicircular canals, embedded in the temporal bone of the skull. The three canals are oriented at right angles to each other. Their normal function is to provide a sense of one's spatial orientation: of which way is up. Without them, a person cannot readily keep his balance, and without this sense of balance, man, a two-legged animal, is in serious trouble. Since the semicircular canals share the same fluid that bathes the nerve of hearing within the cochlea, they offered surgeons an enticing opportunity to circumvent the effects of otosclerosis. It might be possible, they reasoned, to make a new window, or fenestra, in the wall of one of the canals by approaching it surgically via the same route used in performing a mastoidectomy. In this way, they would avoid the risks of penetrating the eardrum while providing the surgeon with a clear view of what he was doing.

Success came slowly. Passow, a German surgeon, tried making a window in the cochlea's base in 1897. He covered it with the membrane that normally covers the bone, and the patient recovered his hearing for a few days. Then in 1899 a Swedish otologist named B. Floderus who wanted to minimize the danger to the cochlear nerve decided to use the techniques of mastoidectomy in order to reach the rearmost semicircular canal. Again hearing was improved; again the result was temporary. In 1913 an Englishman, G. J. Jenkins, made an opening in the horizontal canal, which is easier to reach. He covered the fenestra with a skin graft. Once more hearing improved very dramatically, only to fall off to the old level of deafness or even worse.

During the 1920's, a Swedish and a French surgeon gradually improved the technique of fenestration: Gunnar Holmgren established the principle of using magnification and of operating in an absolutely clean, aseptic field. Maurice Sourdille refined Holmgren's operation into a meticulous, two-stage procedure. But none of these attempts achieved much popularity, even though Holmgren's and Sourdille's techniques were much more successful than any of their predecessors'.

The man who made fenestration a successful *and* an accepted surgical treatment for otosclerotic deafness was an American named Julius Lempert. He was a New Yorker with whom most American otolaryngologists wanted to have as little to do as possible. Born and raised in the ghetto on New York's East Side, he was a thorn in the side of the respectable members of his profession. He was smart; he was acquisitive; he was contemptuous of the comfortable morality of his more successful colleagues. And he was a Jew. He was also Napoleonically short of stature and showed his Bonapartist character by organizing and running a highly lucrative surgical practice out of his own private hospital in Manhattan. He wore obviously very expensive clothes, collected obviously very expensive art, patronized New York's most expensive speak-easies, and rode about New York in the tonneau of the biggest limousine money could buy, driven by a Hollywood version of a chauffeur.

Until he devised a simpler, one-stage fenestration operation based on Sourdille's laborious two-stage technique, he was considered to be on the fringes of what respectable members of the profession regarded as ethical behavior. Perhaps this was because of allegations that he was not above splitting his surgical fees with the lowlier practitioners from Brooklyn, the Bronx, and the Lower East Side who referred patients to him in droves. But the disapproval of more exalted physicians did not prevent them from coming to his first little seven- or eight-bed hospital on 57th Street, crowded with patients from all over town, to consult on a difficult or complicated case.

One of these regular consultants was my mentor, Dr. Isadore Friesner. Whenever Dr. Lempert encountered a par-

ticularly troublesome mastoid case, he would call in Dr. Friesner to help him out, which Dr. Friesner gladly did, of course,
especially since he always collected a very adequate consultation fee. Nor did their qualms prevent other ear surgeons from
coming later to Lempert's new and far more elegant "Endaural Hospital" on East 74th Street in order to learn his ingenious technique of creating the "fenestra nov-ovalis." They
came in groups of eight and each unhesitatingly paid a sizable
fee for a six-week course, practicing on cadavers supplied by
Dr. Lempert, and observing him perform surgery on the living.

Despite Dr. Friesner's earlier association with Dr. Lempert as a consultant, he was adamant in forbidding the attending surgeons on the otologic service at Mount Sinai Hospital
to learn the Lempert fenestration technique. Perhaps this was
because Dr. Friesner himself feared that his junior men might
benefit unduly by learning to perform an operation that he,
Dr. Friesner, could not or would not perform. Or perhaps he
simply felt embarrassed about the earlier relationship he had
had with Dr. Lempert. Naturally, his juniors did not wish to
offend Dr. Friesner, so they stayed away from Dr. Lempert's
hospital and ignored his operation studiously.

The time came when I decided that I would have to
learn this important new technique whether my chief—who
was also my associate in practice—liked it or not. Dr. Lempert
was most cordial. Of course he would be glad to show Dr.
Friesner's colleague the procedure. In fact, he would be happy
to have me take the entire course without fee. For the next
months I spent every spare moment with Dr. Lempert, watching him operate, asking questions, practicing the operation on
cadavers in the basement of the Endaural Hospital, going back
to the operating room to note the ways in which this immensely skillful little man with the big head and torso and
the stumpy arms and legs overcame a thousand difficulties in
order to relieve otosclerotic deafness. But if Dr. Lempert's

generosity to me was motivated by the hope that I could persuade Dr. Friesner to come and observe the operation, thereby putting his blessing upon it, it was a vain hope. My senior not only refused to go to the hospital on 74th Street but persisted in his unremitting disapproval of those who did insist on studying the fenestration nov-ovalis.

The name was a good one, because Lempert's method (see Figure 3, p. 55) made it possible to construct a new oval window—about 1 millimeter wide by 3 millimeters long—simulating the dimensions of the natural opening in which the footplate rests. Because of its size, Lempert's fenestra had a far better chance of remaining open, unlike openings made elsewhere in the semicircular canals; but that was not the only reason why his operation came to be hailed as the answer to otosclerotic hearing loss. There were failures, of course. He thoroughly investigated the causes and concluded that bone dust left in the new opening, rough edges around the window, failure to polish the surface of the bone before creating the fenestra, and other important minutiae of the operative procedure all added up to stimulating regrowth of bone that closed the fenestra and cut off the patient's newly restored hearing. One by one, he found the correct technical answers to each problem, so that at last he was able to declare: "Fenestration does not pretend to cure the lesion of otosclerosis in the region of the oval window but it can and does cure clinical otosclerosis by rendering it symptom-free."

Well, not quite. Fenestration restores a great deal of the hearing lost as a consequence of fixation of the stapes, but the patient still has an average loss of about 25 decibels for the frequencies in the range of human speech. This is so vastly better than barely being able to hear at all, that most patients and their surgeons were delighted with the result. And besides, it was for years "the only game in town"; either you came to New York to Julius Lempert or you went to one of his disciples, like the eminent George E. Shambaugh, Jr., in Chicago, H. P. House in Los Angeles, or Philip Meltzer in Boston, to mention only three out of scores of students.

Julius Lempert shared some of the personal qualities of Thomas Alva Edison and Henry Ford: inventiveness, perspicacity, and a terrible hunger for acceptance, for the esteem, if not the love, of his peers. The secret of Lempert's success was his tenacity and sure judgment in selecting all that was scientifically sound in the pioneering work of Holmgren and Sourdille, while discarding the rest. And he took infinite pains to perfect the technique they had outlined. In other words, Dr. Lempert was a perfectionist. And this was just as well, for every fenestration surgeon must be a perfectionist. The essence of his craft lies in the fact that he must always seek to circumvent nature. Nature is his enemy, because the body, particularly the bone, naturally responds to surgical intervention by mustering its regenerative powers. Nature closes wounds if she can. But the wound that Julius Lempert deliberately made in the bone of the horizontal semicircular canal must not close. Nature must somehow be prevented from shutting the window that he opened to sound, or else the patient's recuperative powers would cruelly deprive him of the hearing he had regained.

In a hundred painstaking experimental variations of the technique of fenestration, Lempert evolved the definitive method of restoring hearing by by-passing the encrusted and immobilized stapes. It worked, and gradually his colleagues in the specialty began to recognize him for what he was: one of the great pioneers in surgery of the ear and, moreover, one of the most skillful ear surgeons it would ever be their privilege to observe. They came from all over the country—from all over the world—to learn how to do the Lempert fenestration.

At the height of his fame, Julius Lempert found himself sought out by the rich and famous around the globe, admired and honored at last by the most distinguished members of his profession, by the American Medical Association, the American Laryngological, Rhinological and Otological Society, the American Otological Society, and, as time passed, by distinguished foreign societies representing the otologic specialty in their lands. He received degrees, gold medals, awards, certificates of honor. Above all, he won the sincerest form of professional acclaim: the unabashed demand of his fellow ear surgeons that he teach them how to open a window of sound in the horizontal semicircular canal of men and women with otosclerosis.

Yet it was all as ashes in his mouth. Despite wealth, fame, and the genuine admiration of peers, Lempert continued to live more in the desperate, frustrating past than in the glowing present. He worked incessantly, earning fabulous fees for his skillful performance of the fenestration procedure and more thousands of uninflated 1940 dollars each year in fees paid him by the surgeons who took his six-week course in fenestration surgery.

But progress in science is inexorable. New methods are developed. Better, less dangerous, less traumatic ways are devised to deal effectively with a given medical problem. As it happened, it was my fate to be the one who would find a way not only to render the lesion of otosclerosis "symptom-free" but to do precisely what Dr. Lempert conceded that fenestration does not do: to "cure the lesion of otosclerosis in the region of the oval window." Others have carried my work further, and I know that as surely as the sun rises, another man will some day render my work obsolete, relegating it to an interesting technique occasionally resorted to when better, still undiscovered techniques are not suited to a particular case.

This is what happened to fenestration surgery when stapes mobilization was finally recognized by the profession as the technique of choice in most instances.

But to Dr. Lempert, the new surgery was anathema. He refused to acknowledge it, refused to practice it, refused to have anything to do with its discoverer, though he had known me well and had patiently taught me his own superb surgical techniques. The last time I saw him was heartbreaking. The occasion was the American Medical Association annual meeting in 1956. Anxious to acquaint as many American doctors as possible with stapes mobilization, I had prepared a scientific exhibit which showed exactly how the procedure was performed. Visitors could look into the ear canals of cadavers whose heads I had prepared and mounted to demonstrate each stage of the operation. Drawings and other visual aids supplemented this stark method of presentation.

To my great delight, the exhibit won the Hektoen Gold Medal for originality and excellence of presentation. But what mattered even more to me was that it drew hundreds of professional visitors, most of whom learned for the first time that there was a new way to cope with otosclerotic deafness.

One day during the meeting, I left the exhibit briefly. When I returned, there was Dr. Lempert. He stood perhaps 20 feet from it, but it was obvious that, however great his aversion to this unsettling development in ear surgery, his curiosity had overcome it. Or so I thought. I went over to him, but he made no move to greet me or shake hands. I stopped, bewildered and rather taken aback. The sudden rush of pleasure I had felt at his appearance died as I realized with a sinking heart that Dr. Lempert had deliberately waited until I was absent to make an appearance. Still, I was determined to say something to him that would, I hoped, appeal to his instincts as a scientist and an innovator.

"Dr. Lempert, you would do me great honor," I began, "if you would permit me to show you my exhibit."

He said nothing, and it became a terrible effort to go on. Nevertheless, I persisted: "The whole world knows you as the greatest ear surgeon of our times. We all respect you for what you have accomplished, and I only was hoping that you would find my contribution of some merit too."

He stood there, saying not a word, his hands thrust into the side pockets of his jacket, his eyes seemingly looking right through me. It was as if he had heard nothing, seen nothing. Then abruptly he turned and walked away quickly.

I have always profoundly regretted that Dr. Lempert could not adapt to this revolutionary development in surgery for conductive hearing loss. If he had brought his remarkable mind and fantastic surgical skills to bear on the problem, he would surely have made many vitally important contributions to the new technique. But it was not to be. Embittered, he turned his back on it and me. This brilliant man had been so hurt by life itself, so devastated, apparently, that he soon began to deteriorate physically and mentally. In a few years, he was dead.

# Of Abandonment and Brotherhood

------------------------------------------------------------------

Julius Lempert's rejection of my work was the product of forces within him that he could not control; but at the time, I experienced it acutely as a personal rejection. I thought of him and of Isadore Friesner as professional fathers to whom I owed whatever knowledge and skills I possessed. They had provided me with the means to develop a wonderful new curative operation for certain kinds of deafness. Now Dr. Lempert had turned away from me in bitterness and resentment. I felt utterly abandoned.

This was a familiar feeling. When I was a child, the fear of being abandoned swept over me often. We lived in the ghetto of Syracuse, New York. I was the fourth of five children, and we were very poor. My father sold crockery in a desultory sort of way, peddling it from house to house. Sometimes he would return with most of his wares unsold. My mother would then load it all into the baby buggy and go down the street, trying to sell enough of the stuff to our neighbors, most of whom were as poor as we were, to scrape together the money for a meal or two. Sometimes she left me to go selling. Her absence terrified me.

My mother was a strong woman, strong in her mind, in her convictions, and, despite chronic asthma, strong of body. She was a little wisp of a woman, but she ran the family. She was Commander in Chief. Her recurrent attacks of asthma were terribly frightening. I remember watching her gasp for breath. Her eyes would bulge, she would wheeze, and her skin would turn an ashen gray as the attack worsened. It seemed to me that she would surely suffocate. I was afraid she would die before the doctor could get there and give her an injection to relieve the bronchospasm. These attacks recurred and recurred. As I grew older, I realized that they would continue to plague her, unless something were done. I resolved to be the one to do that something. I would become a doctor, find the cure for asthma, and forever lift this burden from my mother.

But another abandonment, a painful one, inadvertently deflected me from medicine for a time. As a youngster, I worked as a delivery boy for a grocer named Johnnie Brachis. At first he would pay me at the end of each week, but then a Saturday came when he said: "Sam, I don't have quite enough this week. I'll pay you for this week and next week come next Saturday, all right?" That was all right with me. I knew Johnnie and liked him. If he needed the money, I was glad to let him keep it until next Saturday, especially since I was saving the cash. I thought it was just as good to save it with Johnnie.

The next Saturday came and Johnnie made the same suggestion. He would just keep what he owed me and pay me the *next* Saturday for all three weeks, all right? I agreed.

Every Saturday, Johnnie would say the same thing. It began to mount up, but I went along with it. It occurred to me that Johnnie might have some other reason for holding out my wages, but my family kept reassuring me. Johnnie wouldn't do anything wrong.

"Mr. Brachis is a fine man," Mom said. "He needs the money right now, but he'll pay you, all right. Don't ask him for it, Simkha. Don't you go bothering Mr. Brachis."

The store was close to school. Inevitably there came a Monday when I saw a sign in the window. The store was closed. Padlocked by the sheriff. I ran over and peered into the darkened room. Johnnie Brachis was gone. Every day I stopped in front of the lonely sign, hoping against hope that Johnnie would somehow have reappeared. My heart was sick. It was very lonely. The money—well, the money was important, but it wasn't really uppermost in my mind when I pressed my face against the glass window.

"Poor Johnnie!" I thought. "What's happened to him? Why did he do this? Why did he do this to me?"

One afternoon as I stared morosely at the empty shelves inside, remembering the bustle of business, remembering where all the goods Johnnie stocked were supposed to go, a horse and buggy drove up. I looked around. It was Mr. Murphy, the butter man. He got down and read the sign in silence.

"What happened to Johnnie?" he asked. Mr. Murphy sold tubs of butter to Johnnie and had seen me around the store.

"I don't know, Mr. Murphy," I said. "He's disappeared. He's run away, and nobody knows where he's gone to."

"Not likely he'll be back," Mr. Murphy said knowingly. "Say, boy! He owe you any money?"

"Yes, sir. Two and a half dollars a week for six weeks."

"Well, I guess we're in the same boat," Mr. Murphy said. "Owed me money too. All right, me lad, I'm going downtown to see my lawyer. You hop in the buggy with me and you can talk to him too. Come along with you, now."

We drove down to the commercial section of Syracuse. Mr. Murphy hitched his horse to the curb in front of an office building and took me upstairs with him to his lawyer's office. The lawyer, whose name I have forgotten but never his kindness, was a huge, big-boned, white-haired man. Mr. Murphy explained the situation. The lawyer sat at his rolltop desk and made notes as I told my story.

"Son," he said, "we'll get your money for you. Don't worry about it."

Getting my wages back proved a little more complicated than that. Weeks passed. Then the lawyer sent me a note telling me to come to his office on a weekday morning. I got excused from school and went downtown. Together the lawyer, Mr. Murphy, and I walked around the corner to the courthouse. He had me take the witness stand and asked me questions to bring out the facts, and then the judge asked questions.

"You're going to get your money, all right, Sam," the lawyer said, and sure enough, some weeks later he sent me another note to come to his office after school.

When I arrived, he handed me my $15.

"This is the money Johnnie owed me," I said. "Now, what about your money?"

"No, I don't want any money," he said, smiling down at me. "You were right to ask, but you earned that money and I'm glad you got it. So you keep it."

I thanked him. The money meant a great deal, but the lawyer's kindliness and interest in me meant even more. He had reached out his hand to me when I needed help, when, in fact, I wouldn't have known how to get help.

"Sam, what are you going to be when you grow up?" he asked.

"I'm going to be a doctor."

"Well, that's fine, that's fine," he said. "Tell you what, though, why don't you come to the courthouse with me sometime soon and watch and listen to the things that go in the court. You might like that. You might like it even better than doctoring."

After what he had done for me, I could hardly have refused, just out of politeness; but that was the least of it. This powerful man who knew judges and politicians and lawyers thought of me as potentially an attorney like himself. The thought stirred me. I looked at myself in the mirror and saw a new person. The face was the same, but a man was emerging, a man who would move out of the narrow little world of Grape Street one way or another. It was all very well to dream of becoming a doctor, but I hated the sight of blood and was appalled at the thought of having to face sickness and death directly, to touch dead people, to do all those things I dimly realized a doctor would have to do. The law and its practitioners began to take on more and more appeal.

Under my new friend's guidance, I started to attend trials. I stared at the black-robed judge, at the jury, at the witnesses. Above all, the attorneys for the plaintiff and the defendant enthralled me. The District Attorney was my hero when he presented his case, but the defense attorney immediately captured my loyalty when he took over. The whole setting impressed me profoundly: the grandeur of the big courthouse; the judge in his robes; the oil paintings of solemn-looking great men; the polished oaken railings. It seemed to me that I had entered a veritable heavenly place of justice. Such quiet prevailed, such decorum. And the language! "May it please the Court . . . If Your Honor please . . . Respectfully except from Your Honor's ruling . . . Offer to prove . . . Object to that, Your Honor, on the ground that . . ." No rough talk here! No, sir!

In no time I became a thoroughgoing court buff. I picked my own cases to attend. Whole vacations passed in the courtroom. I would identify myself with the plaintiff first, and then with the defendant, especially when I thought he was getting the worst of it, but then if the plaintiff wasn't doing too well, I would be sorry for him too. I was terribly offended when I thought a witness was lying and another man being hurt as a consequence. I wanted to get after this fellow who was perjuring himself and make him pay for the harm he was doing by lying. As a high-school student, I was learning about such American ideals as equal justice under law and other rights that citizens were supposed to have. But as I followed trial after trial, I began to realize that what I thought of as right, decent, and just was not what I always saw in the courtroom. Witnesses lied; lawyers played tricks; even the judge was not always absolutely fair. Of course, it never occurred to me that a judge could be corrupt, that he could be "fixed," that he could be hiding outright prejudice behind his robes. Why, that would be like imagining that God was fixed!

In my eyes, the system was as fair and honest as the mind of man could make it. It was men's frailty and venality that caused all the trouble. Justice would be served in the courtroom, if only the schemes, lies, plots, and plans of bad men could be exposed. Sometimes an able lawyer's cross-examination would catch a witness in a contradiction. The witness would squirm. He would twist and turn in the chair and mumble his answers, and the triumphant lawyer would call on him to "speak up so His Honor and the gentlemen of the jury can hear your answer; you're not ashamed of the answer, are you?"

"Objection!"

"Sustained."

Scenes like this delighted and infuriated me; delighted me because I enjoyed seeing the discomfiture of the false witness; infuriated me, because even to me it was obvious that he was not going to be punished for lying. Lying witnesses got away with it. The judge, the attorneys, all these sophisticated great men *expected* some witnesses to lie, and had no intention of giving them their just deserts. They were not going to be punished and I knew it, and the thought outraged me. How could people be like that? The reality of it rudely violated my ideal of how people should behave. In my family, poor as we

were, hard-pressed as we were, I never witnessed a single act
of dishonesty.

By the time I had finished high school, I had decided to
become a lawyer. I would fight for the truth. I would be able
to see through the liars and cheats. I would see that they were
punished. I would protect the innocent and the wronged
against them.

Just about this time, a famous trial took place in Syracuse.
Former President Theodore Roosevelt was suing a man named
Barnes, who was editor of an Albany newspaper, for libel. I
suppose the venue of the case had been moved to Syracuse because the Albany paper had so much influence in that city.
Of course, I was determined to see these giants locked in
combat, and as an experienced court buff, I prevailed upon the
bailiff to let me into the packed courtroom.

"I'm going to be a lawyer myself," I told him. Whether
he believed me or not, he let me slip past the tall oaken doors.

I found a place to stand near the witness chair. There, so
close I could almost touch him, was Teddy, the great man
himself, just as I had seen him pictured in the newspapers, his
eyeglasses and teeth gleaming. The only other time I had seen
him was when he spoke, shouting at a great distance to a huge
crowd. It was thrilling beyond the telling! Here was history
being made, right in the presence of Sam Rosen.

Johnnie had abandoned me, but Mr. Murphy's lawyer
had taken his place in my heart. You could help the poor and
defenseless by being a lawyer, I decided, just as well as you
could by becoming a doctor.

My older brothers and my sister had never even considered
going to college, but they were determined to see that I went.
We had practically no money, but they and my parents and I
scrimped and saved. I worked vacations, summers, and weekends. When I finished my first year in the school of liberal
arts, I announced to them that I was going to enter law school.

It was a wonderful experience. The fine differences in semantics fascinated me, the delicate shades of meaning in phrases. The neatness of it, the orderliness and logic of the whole discipline attracted me. So did the precision of the rules of procedure, of evidence, of motions. You couldn't stray from the beaten path here: everything was carefully mapped out.

Criminal law interested me especially; business law, contracts, torts, estates less so. I especially relished the idea of thinking a complex situation through carefully. Was this judge correct in his opinion? Or was the higher court more correct?

For the rest of my life I have remembered Mr. Murphy's lawyer saying: "All right, now, let's sit down and get all the facts, all the facts." Facts were what mattered, not a person's conclusions or opinions. If you had the facts, opinions would have to yield to them; conclusions would have to follow from them. I didn't know it then, but this is as true in clinical medicine and in research as it is in any other discipline worthy of the name. In those two years I learned irrevocably that where an opinion, a diagnosis, a prognosis, a conclusion does not fit the facts, the opinion must yield, not the facts. Facts exist. An opinion is merely held, until the weight of factual evidence forces the holder to change it or to be left, like poor Julius Lempert, clinging to the past, turning his back on the future.

Decisions, however, are not always based on conscious knowledge. I know this from much personal experience. In 1919, after I had completed a third of my law studies, I woke one summer morning in my room at home on Grape Street, knowing that something momentous had happened to me during the night. I came downstairs to the kitchen and sat at the table while my mother bustled about preparing breakfast.

"Mom," I said embarrassedly, "I don't know why I'm going to law school. I've always wanted to be a doctor, and I still do. I want to quit law and go to the medical college."

Perhaps I half expected her to point out that I had wasted a whole year and much dearly earned money. Certainly I thought my brothers would say that it was hard enough to send me through college once without having to put up with my indecisiveness. No such thing. They were firmly behind my decision to go into medicine, even though it meant supporting my education for longer than they had planned.

I soon knew that I had made the right decision. Medical school fascinated me in a way that the law had not. Medicine might be less precise—and that was putting it mildly!—but it offered a direct opportunity to help others who were in trouble. By comparison, the law was just another way of making a living at the expense of people in trouble or in the service of the business establishment. Since I was not temperamentally suited to either role, it was just as well that I got out of the study of law as soon as I did.

But it was not to be the last time that a change of circumstance or a change of mind brought about a change in my plans. As a result, after my internship at Mount Sinai Hospital in 1923 there was another family conference in Syracuse.

"I have been offered an attractive residency in the big city, followed by an association with Dr. Friesner," I explained. Then I put it up to them.

"I know you all expect me to come back to Syracuse to practice," I said, "and that's what I will do if you tell me to."

"Sam," my mother said—as always, she was chairman of the board, "you have to do what is best for you."

"But after all you've all done for me, how can I—"

"Sam!" It was one of my brothers. "You don't understand. We're doing this for ourselves too. We get a big kick out of seeing you move up in the world. That's what we're getting out of it."

It was a tremendous relief to hear this. All through medical school and internship I had grown more and more uneasy about practicing internal or general medicine. As an intern I had been in charge of two wards comprising about sixty beds. Two, three, sometimes four times a day I made rounds, examining patients, ordering tests, trying to get more facts, more data on which to base a more accurate diagnosis and more effective treatment. So many were beyond my help, beyond the help even of the most skilled medical men on the hospital staff. Medicine really had nothing to offer many severely ill patients in those days, except the best possible conditions under which their natural defenses against disease might suffice to conquer their ailments. Too often that was not enough, and we would have to watch a man or woman lying there slowly succumbing to disease.

Sometimes things turned out more happily. A young man in his twenties was admitted. He had a high fever, and was delirious. Examining him, I soon concluded that he had lobar pneumonia, often a fatal illness in those days. He grew steadily worse. One night, I was so concerned about him that I watched him through the night, even though there was absolutely nothing I could do for him. Toward morning a crisis was reached. His temperature dropped precipitately, his delirium disappeared. In a matter of days he was shakily getting to his feet and soon he was discharged. Several years later, I hailed a cab, and the driver said: "Hiya, doc! Get in." It was my former patient, strong, husky, and in glowing health. He took me to my destination but refused to accept the fare.

"You saved my life, Dr. Rosen," he said. "How can I take money from you? Forget it, will ya?"

I hadn't saved his life. He had saved his own. In vain I explained that to him, but he brushed it aside. I was just not taking the credit I ought to have, he said. He absolutely refused to take my money.

As my internship progressed, I found myself on the ear, nose, and throat service for several months. Almost at once I knew I had finally found my place in medicine. The surgery in this specialty was especially satisfying to me, because it required a meticulousness and a precision that surgery in roomier parts of the human anatomy did not demand. Above all, there were so many things one could do for patients. You knew for certain that a tonsillectomy, or a mastoidectomy, for instance, would definitely improve the patient's health or would ward off more serious, perhaps fatal, complications.

Furthermore, it soon became evident even to me, as it was to the chief of the service, that I had real promise as a surgeon. One day I assisted the chief, Dr. Friesner, in a mastoidectomy. He let me carry out more than the merely routine parts of the operation. Afterwards, as we dressed, Dr. Friesner asked: "What are you planning to specialize in, Sam?"

"Why general practice or internal medicine, I guess, Dr. Friesner."

He must have known that I was not all that certain.

"You ought to think about otology," he said. "If you decide in favor of it, I will be glad to have you as a resident here. It could lead to an association with me in practice, if everything works out all right."

# Of Love and Paternalism

-----------------------------------------------------------------------------

In two more years I had completed my residency. True to his
word, Dr. Friesner took me into practice with him and saw
that I was appointed as attending surgeon on the ear, nose, and
throat service at Mount Sinai. The years of scrimping and
saving were over. I was now a skilled young "Park Avenue"
specialist, associated with one of New York's most distinguished
—and affluent!—practitioners.

Fortunately for me, Dr. Friesner did not particularly care
to perform many of the surgical procedures that our practice
required. That was undoubtedly one reason why he offered me
an association with him, especially since he had also concluded
that my competence as a surgeon was more than adequate.
He made no secret of his opinion of my abilities, and of course
the judgment of a chief of service is not ignored by his colleagues. I began to get referrals. Everyone quite naturally assumed that I was destined eventually to take over not only his
very lucrative practice but his position as chief.

I was a devoted pupil when it came to medicine and surgery, but a gulf separated us in every other aspect of life. Dr. Friesner was ultra-conservative. I had no quarrel with his philosophical outlook, except that I simply did not share it, and even in practice our paths diverged when our basic outlook on life was involved. He was, for instance, a past master at the art of examining and questioning a patient. Nothing was left to guesswork. Every possible clue to the nature and cause of the patient's complaints was searched for. It was an experience to watch and listen as he methodically took the most detailed of histories and then conducted the most thorough physical examination. He "got all the facts," and only then did he weigh the accumulated evidence and arrive at his diagnosis.

Not only did I admire his diagnostic skill, I sought earnestly to emulate it, and my "wasted" years in law school stood me in good stead. But, once a diagnosis had been made, Dr. Friesner and I parted company in the way we related to our patients. Dr. Friesner told them as little as possible. He was a big, jolly, fat man. He had an endless repertoire of jokes that he told to put patients at ease. He felt he had neither the time, the patience, nor the desire to explain things to the patient. Why bother? He knew what was good for them and that was enough. If you explain something to the patient, the chances are he will ask you some damn fool question, he thought, and of course he was right. Patients have the absurd notion that what is happening to them is happening to *them* and is therefore something they are entitled to understand. Dr. Friesner's view of this was that the physician's white coat should protect him from such "nonsense." Of course, he had a lot of company. Many doctors adopted this attitude and still do, partly because they really are terribly hard-pressed for time, but also because it spares them the annoyance of having to answer difficult or embarrassing questions, the truthful answers to many of which are "We don't know," or "I'm afraid medical science has no answer to this problem as yet."

For a while, I tried imitating my mentor's bedside and consulting-room manner, but it didn't suit my personality. I liked to listen to patients and talk to them. I discovered that to me they weren't "mastoids" or "tonsils" or "sinuses"; they were people in trouble. It turned out that, if I listened and questioned and answered long enough, as often as not the patient would come up with the essential clue to what was wrong with him. This took time, but perhaps in the long run it saved even more, and in addition, spared the patient the expense and discomfort that result when the wrong diagnosis and the wrong treatment are first adopted. Besides, communication is so important. It is part of the treatment. If an atmosphere of warmth and trust develops in the patient-physician relationship, both are better off, no matter what the disease. Patients do, of course, put their confidence in noble-looking, gray-haired doctors, but their trust rests on shaky foundations. The patient rightly feels that he has lost control of his destiny. His fate is in hands other than his own. As long as all goes well, he remains confident, but the slightest setback can destroy his security. The fight goes out of him, perhaps even the will to live, and when that happens, an impossible burden is placed on the doctor.

There was one situation, however, in which I was not able to practice what I have been preaching. I could never tell a patient or his next of kin that his case was hopeless, not even when I was as certain as anyone could be that this was so. Indeed, there is no real certainty. Life is uncertain, chancy, unpredictable. So is death.

During my internship a patient on my ward proved to have carcinoma of the lung. Both of his lungs were riddled with the cancer. There was no hope. Surgery could do nothing for him—you can't take out *both* lungs. Radium treatment palliated it a little, perhaps, but we had to tell his family that he just had no chance. Understandably, his family decided to take him home to die. Three years later, the man came into Mount Sinai's out-patient clinic with some trivial complaint. Not a trace of cancer. We rushed for his medical records, his X-rays, his bedside charts. There was absolutely no question of the diagnosis, yet here he was, hale and hearty. At a medical conference later, his case was presented to some two hundred doctors, not, unfortunately, so much as an object lesson in the folly of predicting death as an example of an unexplained miracle. Yet we know that this happens, more often, probably, than we suppose. Even cancer sometimes yields to the amazing capacity of the organism to overcome disease. A whole text-book is devoted to instances of proven cases of cancer that later spontaneously regressed and disappeared.

Once again, it is the patient who is the fact, whereas the prognosis of even the most distinguished physician is still only an opinion, and an opinion can only be an estimate of the meaning of whatever facts we have been able to uncover. It is not the fact itself.

Not long after this incident, something happened that changed the whole course of my life. A young college girl was brought by train to New York and by ambulance to the hospital. She was desperately ill, and her parents, although not wealthy, were both successful New York lawyers. They were members of an aristocratic Sephardic Jewish family, and they knew and had unlimited confidence in Isadore Friesner. Consultants were called in at once. The girl, Alice van Dernoot, was obviously in critical condition. She had dangerously high fever, and blood tests indicated an infection somewhere was the immediate cause. We decided that in all likelihood it was in her sinuses. Within the hour of her arrival, the patient was in surgery. I opened and drained her sinuses. They were badly infected. The immediate danger was now lessened, but the girl continued to be gravely ill. She had septicemia. Her kidneys became involved. Consultants came and went. Her parents sent for her older sister, Helen, who was attending Wellesley College.

Because she had originally been assigned to me, Alice was my patient. As always with a gravely ill patient, I kept a careful eye on the situation, visiting her room frequently, talking to her and to her parents and sister. Distinguished consultants came, examined her, and called the relatives outside. They shook their heads. The unfortunate young woman, they said, would probably not recover. Even though I thought they were probably right, their saying so angered me. I didn't want to hold out false hope, but I knew there was always some bit of hope one can offer. When the big men left, I told Helen and her parents about the patient with lung cancer.

"Don't give up hope," I said. "We're just doctors, not God. We can't predict the future. We don't know everything about any disease or any patient. She's very, very sick, but that doesn't mean she can't make it. I don't know whether she will or not, but I'm damned if I will give up on it, and don't you, either."

Perhaps the parents didn't take the young doctor too seriously, but the older sister did. She hung around Alice's room, running errands for the nurses, and just being generally useful. It was a nice thing to see, and I got in the habit of dropping in every time I went on rounds and then again in the evening. Helen was the kind of girl I had only seen at a distance, stepping into or out of Pierce-Arrow limousines, or Stutz Bearcats, emerging from fancy Fifth Avenue stores laden with packages, going arm in arm with well-dressed young brokers into speak-easies where an evening of eating, drinking, and entertainment cost as much as I made in a month! She was everything that I was not, cultured, elegant, but here she was looking after her sister and keeping her parents' spirits up. I liked her. I found I could talk to her and that she could both talk and listen to me, even though most of the men she knew and went out with were, in those years of crazy prosperity, rich men's sons who lived on unearned income and talked about "the market" and parties and a whole world quite foreign to me.

Slowly, by inches, Alice got better. The consultants looked pleased and forgot about their grim forebodings. The van Dernoots began to smile.

"You must come to see us, Dr. Rosen," they said. "Alice thinks the world of you, of course."

They may have had some notions about me and Alice, but it was Helen I came to see, Helen whom I took out, though not to the fancy speak-easies she was accustomed to, and Helen to whom I finally mustered the nerve to propose.

We were married on November 26, 1928, at the van Dernoot apartment in the Hyde Park Hotel. My brothers and sister came to the wedding, but my mother was too ill and my father stayed with her in Syracuse. Helen had never met them. After the wedding we took a train to Syracuse. It was all strange to Helen. The tracks ran right down the main street. We took a taxi to visit my parents. I remember Helen asking me what the "incense" was in my parents' house. It was a patent-medicine fulminating powder that my mother thought helped her asthma. We stayed that night in a hotel, visited my parents once more, and left for our honeymoon at Virginia Beach.

The Friesners were delighted with the marriage. Mrs. Friesner insisted that Helen come to visit often. They wanted literally to take us completely into their family, and even went to the point of asking me to change my name to Friesner. Of course we wouldn't consider such a thing. To me it would have been a repudiation of all that my family had done to help me become a doctor and to find my place in life. I tried to explain this to Dr. Friesner, and I like to think he accepted it as graciously as he could, but it was the beginning of what grew to be an increasing strain in our relationship. Helen and I insisted on living our own lives. We did not intend to limit our interests to medicine or our friendships to physicians. We liked some of them well enough, but we wanted to be a part of the larger world, the world of music, art, politics, everything that was going on.

The Depression began just a year after we were married. My practice nevertheless grew and prospered, but all around us we saw suffering, breadlines, legless veterans selling apples. Most of my colleagues didn't seem to notice, unless they became aware of the problem of some particular patient. To Helen and me this shocking poverty in a land of plenty made no sense. Helen had voted for Herbert Hoover in 1928 while I voted for Al Smith, mostly because I always identify with the underdog. In 1932 we agreed on Franklin D. Roosevelt. He spoke our language. Helen began to be active in support of candidates like Roosevelt, Mayor Fiorello LaGuardia, and other liberals and reformers. The Friesners definitely did not like it. How could we vote for "that man"? How could Helen, the wife of a rising young otologist, go out on the streets with a flag, a stepladder, and a megaphone and make speeches and distribute socialistic-sounding literature? It wasn't right, it wasn't proper. Why don't you say something to her, Sam?

I don't recall whether the Friesners knew, or even whether I told them, that not only was I proud of my beautiful, patrician wife's concern for the unemployed, the poor, the people F.D.R. called the "ill-clothed, ill-housed, ill-fed" third of our nation—not only was I proud of her for her involvement, I was involved too. It was I—and when they grew old enough, our daughter and son, Judy and John (whom we called "Friesie" because his middle name was Friesner)—who handed out the "socialistic" literature that explained the New Deal program. Gradually our social relations with the Friesners cooled. Dr.

Friesner and I continued to practice together. When he retired, I rented offices and provided space for him to carry on a reduced schedule in a consulting practice. I owed him that. He was a fine physician and surgeon, and a diagnostician of extraordinary acumen. He taught me much of what I know professionally that is of greatest value. He also taught me indirectly other things, usually by the example of opposites. Early in my practice, he began to turn over patients who needed mastoid surgery but could not afford his fee. I was grateful for these opportunities, and, confident that I was quite as capable as Dr. Friesner, accepted the patients without hesitation. No doubt Dr. Friesner was equally confident that he had done the only right and reasonable thing. Those were the standards of that time in medicine, as, unfortunately, they are still to a great extent in this country. We are supposed to have the finest medical care in the world, but who receives it? Not the poor, not the black, unless they are "fortunate" enough to have a rare or "interesting" condition, one that is useful for teaching and for learning. Looking at this situation in American medicine, the late Dr. Henry E. Sigerist, Professor of the History of Medicine at Johns Hopkins, commented that no man should profit from the misfortunes of his fellow men. Some doctors do. Some doctors know it is wrong, but they are trapped in the system, much as they may deplore it. It is therefore a mistake to blame all doctors for the faults of an outmoded, unworkable system of providing health care to 200 million people.

My colleagues, including Dr. Friesner, of course grew increasingly aware that the Rosens were not quite the nice, conservative, respectable, right-thinking people that they were supposed to be. Helen and I studied sociology at night at Columbia and learned many irreverently stated realities about the American social and political scene. When the civil war in Spain broke out, we were outspoken in our opposition to

Franco and our support of the Republican government. We believed in democracy and thought the democratically elected Loyalist government ought to be supported by the American democracy, not to mention England and France.

We were also aware of what was going on across the Pacific, where imperial Japan had invaded China. Helen became active in the China Aid Council, an organization headed by Madame Sun Yat-sen, whose main function was to purchase medical supplies for shipment behind the Japanese lines to the 8th Route Army.

There were a great many people who felt the same way, even some doctors, but it was not nice to be so open about it. Have your own opinions, but don't "disgrace" the profession and offend the hospital trustees by declaring them out loud. And keep your wife at home, taking care of the kids and arranging dinner parties for your brothers in the profession and their wives. Don't let her run all over the city consorting with Democratic women politicians. That's not what a doctor's wife should be doing.

The doctors of my generation were rather naïve about politics, economics, social problems. I thought surely that many of my colleagues would be sympathetic to Helen's activities in behalf of the Democrats and to my support of her political work. Not so. Most of them didn't like it. Word got around the hospital that Helen was making speeches and with my approval. My colleagues were either silent or openly disapproving. But Roosevelt is for the ordinary guy, like you and me, I would argue. That hardly sat well. They didn't think of themselves as "ordinary guys" and I compounded the error by pointing out how powerless we really were, how fearful we were of the trustees, how careful everyone was of what he said. That only made them angrier, either because they would have liked to say what I was saying but didn't dare, or because they sincerely opposed my ideas.

By the time Dr. Friesner gave up his post as chief of service, it was not very surprising that Dr. Rosen was not appointed to succeed him. Dr. Rosen was a fine surgeon and all that, but, well, he just wasn't the—well, he perhaps did not have the necessary administrative skills for such a responsible post. Something like that. Nothing personal, you understand, but with a man like that, who knows? Why, next year he might be proposing group practice, or a full-time salaried staff, or heaven knows what radical scheme! A more politically and socially acceptable otolaryngologist was appointed.

# Of a Successful Failure

It would not be honest to say that I took this rejection without a qualm. I was hurt. No matter that you know in your heart you are able and deserving and that what has been done to you has been done from motives that do not reflect in any way on your skill, your dedication, or your standards of practice—no matter; the heart is saddened, and unhappy doubts arise in the strongest, most determined souls. Besides, they were, in their way, right: the chiefs have to be acceptable to those who are responsible for the running of a great metropolitan hospital. It takes money, lots of it. Some of it may come from federal grants, some from the city, but millions must come from the city's wealthy men and women. Mount Sinai owes much to philanthropy, especially the generosity of the Guggenheims and the Klingensteins. I don't say that either of these families would have balked at any appointment made by the medical staff of the hospital. I do say that the people whose job it was to attract their interest and solicit their support balked. They are not the kind whose first love is freedom of opinion. Their delight is not in adventure and discovery but in safety and comfort. Helen and I chose to live our own lives, to be free, to speak out and fight for what we believed in. Pericles once said that courage is freedom and freedom is happiness. This is profoundly true. There is a price that you have to pay. The lowest price is doubt, uncertainty, risk. Sometimes the price goes up to character assassination, vilification, and ostracism. And for some, like Martin Luther King, Malcolm X, and others in our time, the price is life itself.

For us, the price was modest. We lost some friends, but we made others who were from different worlds. The escalator to the penthouse stopped, but my practice continued to grow. There were always patients waiting during office hours, and there was always more and more to learn in order to stay abreast of developments in the specialty. I studied, I operated, I read, I treated, I even made house calls.

As time passed, more and more medical men began to think of me as a surgeon to whom their patients could safely be entrusted. Then came World War II. Although I volunteered, a minor disability made me ineligible. Many surgeons went into the armed services, adding immensely to the caseloads of those who remained behind. The war accelerated medical research. The sulfa drugs and then the natural and synthetic antibiotics were developed. It was a therapeutic revolution. I remember vividly a patient on the E.N.T. (ear, nose, and throat) service at Mount Sinai who had a severe mastoid infection complicated by septicemia. He was a shoemaker, elderly and in poor condition. He was so debilitated that I was afraid he would not survive a mastoidectomy. As the assistant attending physician on duty when he was admitted, I ordered a course of sulfa drug therapy, but when my superior, the associate attending physician on the service, came in the next day he was indignant. An operation should be done at once, he said. I disagreed, though I was far from sure. If the new "miracle drug" did not work, I argued, I would still have time to undertake the desperate expedient of operating and, meanwhile, perhaps the infection and the patient's condition might have improved at least a little.

"All right," he said, "have it your own way, Dr. Rosen." But it was obvious that he expected the patient to worsen and die.

For the next several days the interns, residents, and nurses followed the patient's course intently. So did I. It was touch and go. Gradually, the warning signs of high fever and intense sensitivity to pressure on the mastoid bone behind the ear subsided. Finally, he was discharged, cured.

The incident set me to thinking. Here was a dramatic cure of a disease that had appalled physicians since Hippocrates' time. There were obviously going to be fewer and fewer mastoid operations to perform, yet that was my particular skill as a surgeon. What would I be doing when mastoidectomy was no longer an important operation in otology? How could I continue to use my laboriously acquired surgical skills to help patients? Looking at the overall picture, it was increasingly evident to me that ear surgery was going to undergo a major revolution. Instead of being primarily a means to prevent the spread of infection, it was becoming a tool to bring about relief from inherited or acquired disorders of the middle-ear mechanism. Lempert, after all, had found the way to relieve otosclerotic deafness. The operation was tricky, but immensely rewarding, because it did restore useful hearing. This was when I decided that the time had come for me to ignore Dr. Friesner's hostile attitude toward Lempert and his fenestration nov-ovalis and learn how to perform this marvelous new operation.

Even in the hands of a highly skilled surgeon, the operation was a delicate, time-consuming one, lasting four to five hours. In the process, the surgeon has literally to create a new pathway by which sound can reach the inner ear's fluid-filled chamber. To do so, he makes an incision in the skin of the ear canal, exposing the mastoid bone, which he then excavates carefully until he has reached the wall of the horizontal semicircular canal. In the process, he exposes the ossicles

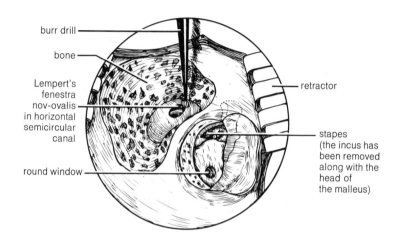

FIGURE 3. *View of surgical field through operating microscope during Lempert's fenestration. The burr has just created the fenestra nov-ovalis.*

(the three middle-ear bones), removing the incus entirely and amputating the parts of the malleus not attached to the eardrum. With a probe, the surgeon then tests the stapes to confirm that it is rigidly fixed in the oval window, for, after all, the purpose of the operation is to circumvent this presumed obstruction to normal sound conduction. If the stapes turns out to be movable, the surgeon assumes that the patient's deafness is not due to otosclerosis and that the fenestration will not restore hearing. But by now he has gone so far that he must continue to make the fenestra. To do so, he must carefully grind down the hard, bony wall of the horizontal canal at its broadest face. At just the right moment he desists and with other instruments detaches and removes an oval piece of the thinned bone to form a new window. Then he covers the artificial opening with a flap of skin that he left attached to the ear canal for just this purpose as he penetrated to the middle ear during the first part of the procedure. If he has taken care to control all bleeding during the operation and especially at this critical juncture, if he is meticulous about aseptic surgical technique, if he has been careful to keep the skin flap and the fenestra's rim free of bone fragments and bone dust, and if he covers the opening in a certain manner devised by Lempert, the patient has a very good chance of recovering adequate enough hearing to obviate the need of a hearing aid—or if he were profoundly deaf, the operation could often restore enough hearing to make the use of a hearing aid successful.

But there are problems, as there are in any surgical procedure. After the operation, the patient must remain in the hospital for two to three weeks. Then the surgeon has to take care of the new pathway down into the middle ear every two or three weeks until it has completely healed. Thereafter, the patient must remember that the labyrinth has been seriously disturbed by the surgery and that he may have severe vertigo if he turns his head abruptly or if he allows cold air to enter the operated ear. Of course he cannot swim. And finally, he must return to the doctor every six months or so to have the cavity cleaned out, since nature has provided no mechanism, as in the normal ear, for the discharge of dead skin cells and foreign material.

All this was a problem for both surgeon and patient, but that did not really matter. For the vast majority of properly selected patients, Lempert's fenestration restored usable hearing. That was what mattered. The patients could hear with the operated ear at least as well as they previously could have only by using a good hearing aid, and of course the quality of their auditory perception was much better than the best hearing aid could provide. Most fenestrated patients get an improvement in hearing to about 20 decibels below the level of a normal young adult. Such a minor loss is hardly noticeable to many patients, and for most of them, this remains relatively stable. For a few, the newly constructed oval window closes over and hearing fades again. For a further very few unlucky ones, the operation sets up an inflammation of the inner ear that may be successfully treated or may, in other cases, result in permanent damage to the nerve with loss of hearing and constant or intermittent vertigo. Fortunately, both kinds of complication are very rare.

All this is accomplished without the elaborate system of drum membrane and leverlike ossicles that I described earlier which acts as the transformer mechanism for the conversion of airborne sound waves into vibrations strong enough to produce waves within the inner ear and movement of the delicate membrane that divides the spiral chamber of the cochlea. How is such a thing possible?

It is possible largely because of the extraordinary range over which the auditory nerve can detect vibrations. The difference between the softest sound that the normal ear can report to the brain and the loudest sound that it can stand without permanent damage is so enormous that scientists use decibels instead of ordinary numbers to express the difference in sound intensity. Zero decibels is defined as the lowest intensity—softer than a whisper—at which the normal young adult can hear sound. Ten db is 10 times louder; 20 db, 100 times louder; 30 db, 1,000 times louder; and so on. A sound with an intensity of 120 db, which will cause the hearer noticeable discomfort, is 1 trillion times louder than the 0 db, or threshold level. Roughly speaking, the decibel levels (using the normal adult o db threshold as the baseline) for various everyday sounds are 30 db for a whisper; 60 db for normal conversation; 80 db for heavy traffic; over 100 db for subway noise. At 120 db one experiences tickling sensations and real discomfort; at 140 db, pain; and at 160 db—the intensity of sound produced by a jet engine with afterburner in an enclosed space—ruinous damage to the ear mechanism results almost at once.

Sound entering the oval window in the normal ear cannot travel through the fluid of the inner ear unless that fluid is free to vibrate. This becomes possible because the inner ear has a second window which bulges outward into the middle ear each time the movement of the footplate in the oval window sets up vibrations in the fluid. We don't have to worry about phase relationships of sound at the oval window and the round window, because the powerful action of the ossicles transforms airborne sound to vibrations that are far stronger than whatever sound arrives by air alone at the round window. Those airborne vibrations could not possibly push hard enough against the round window's membrane to dampen, to any serious extent, the vibration of the fluid in the inner ear.

But suppose the footplate is immobile and the sound has to travel from the new fenestra in the semicircular canal through the cochlea to the round window. The intensity of the sound reaching the fenestra has not been increased by transformer action. Consequently, if the compression wave of sound arrives simultaneously at both the fenestra and the round window, they will exert equal force at each opening, preventing the fluid inside from vibrating and causing no stimulation of the nerve of hearing. If the compression wave arrives at the fenestra just as the rarefaction wave reaches the round window, however, the sound is out of phase, and the round window membrane is free to move, permitting the vibration to pass through the inner ear fluid and to stimulate the nerve.

Nor will fenestration restore hearing if the patient's stapes is, in fact, mobile, instead of being held rigid by otosclerotic growth of bone around the footplate. In such a case, sound enters the fenestra, but it causes the footplate to vibrate, thereby dampening the vibration of the inner-ear fluid and preventing stimulation of the nerve of hearing. Consequently, it is standard practice for most surgeons performing a fenestration to probe the stapes to see that it is fixed.

Usually the stapes is rigid in patients who have been carefully screened by testing and selected for fenestration. Usually, but not always. It is this exception to what was usual that resulted in a new revolution in the surgery of deafness that took place in the 1950's. And since I am the "revolutionist" responsible for the upheaval, I am in a peculiarly favored position to tell how it all came about.

It began on a very ordinary working day. Usually I do my surgery in the mornings, when I am fresh and full of energy. Ear surgery, especially fenestration surgery, requires cool, steady nerves, because the area in which the surgeon must work is so constricted. Furthermore, human beings are not produced on an assembly line with identical, interchangeable parts. Different patients have slightly different anatomical structures. In a cavity like the abdomen, slight differences may not be particularly crucial; but in the middle ear, the slightest variation in the location of, for example, the facial nerve, can spell disaster for the incautious surgeon and his patient. The latter risks emerging from the operating room with half of his face paralyzed at least for a long time, and perhaps partially paralyzed for the rest of his life.

On this particular morning in 1952, I had company. Besides the scrub nurse, there was the late Viennese otologist Dr. Franz Altmann in the operating room with me. He too had become a fenestration surgeon, at Columbia-Presbyterian Medical Center, and was watching me operate. Everything was normal. The patient was a woman whose audiometric tests indicated that she was a perfectly good candidate for a Lempert fenestration: her hearing by bone conduction was practically normal, but the air-conduction curve was far below normal. Presumably her stapes had become fixed in place by otosclerosis.

As always, at the proper point in the operation I exposed the ossicles, cut the joint between incus and malleus, removed the incus, and clipped off the head and neck of the malleus. Then I asked for my probe. Its handle hit my rubber-gloved palm as the nurse placed it there. I prodded the stapes with the end of the probe—and the stapes moved!

"Franz," I said in a low voice, "did you see it move?"

"I'm not sure," he said. "I think so."

We both knew that if the stapes was still mobile, the fenestration would not restore hearing.

It had definitely moved. Feeling a structure move under the pressure of an instrument is more certain evidence than merely looking at the tiny bone while another surgeon handles the instrument.

"Oh Lord," I said. "I'm sure it did."

Since by this time, following Lempert's standard technique, I had already destroyed the patient's normal chain of ossicles from eardrum to oval window, there was no turning back. With a heavy heart, I continued the operation, making the fenestra and employing a new technique I had devised and that Dr. Altmann particularly wanted to observe. Its purpose was to provide perhaps just a little extra insurance against nature's effort to close the fenestra. But all I could really think about was the fact that this woman would almost certainly not benefit from the operation, because her stapes was not rigidly fixed by overgrowth of otosclerotic bone.

After the operation was over, we changed and went down to the cafeteria for a cup of tea. I must have been looking very glum.

"We can't always succeed in what we set out to do," Franz

said kindly in his somewhat formal English. "It could happen to anyone. Surely you have had failures before?"

"You don't think she will get a good result either, do you?" I said tiredly.

"Not if the stapes was mobile, of course not."

"Franz," I asked, "has this ever happened to you?"

He looked thoughtful for a moment and said: "To my certain knowledge, once. And to answer your next question, the operation failed to improve hearing."

We were both terribly depressed by the almost certain prospect that the patient would not benefit from the operation, and we continued to discuss it without coming to any conclusion other than the one all surgeons often come to: that they are only human and that medicine has a long way to go.

Later, when I visited the patient, our fears were confirmed. She had gotten no improvement whatever. I had subjected her to a long, wearisome procedure and, even worse, to the risk, however slight, of serious complications that might adversely affect the nerve of hearing. All for naught. All day the question haunted me. It occurred to me that if it could happen to me and to Franz to his "certain knowledge" at least once, then it must be happening to others. Not every surgeon tested the stapes for mobility during a fenestration operation, so perhaps there were many unreported instances of mobile stapes that caused the procedure to fail.

I spent a restless night. There had to be a way to protect my patients against the time, expense, and risk of undergoing fenestration when the operation could not succeed because the stapes was not rigid. I thought of an operation I had tried in an attempt to halt Ménière's disease by severing the chorda tympani nerve where it passes through the middle ear. The operation was simple. It could be done under local anesthesia, took only about fifteen minutes, and was so minor in its after-effects that the patient could leave the hospital on the following day. Most important, the surgical approach to the middle ear that I had used in this operation was one that allowed me to see the stapes in most cases. It was a surgical approach that Dr. Lempert had devised and had taught me for use in another procedure, tympano-sympathectomy, in which he severed the nerves on the bony wall of the middle ear. Why not use this approach to the middle ear as a preliminary, diagnostic operation to determine how many prospective fenestration patients actually had movable stapes and were therefore not good candidates for the more elaborate operation?

Why not, indeed. I resolved to try this preliminary test in the next one hundred or so consecutive cases. Such a study would provide solid research data for a report to my colleagues on that unanswered question: How many patients who apparently have otosclerotic fixation of the stapes actually have mobile stapes and therefore could not be successfully treated by Lempert's fenestration?

I never got to write the scientific paper I had envisaged. Events moved far too fast and far too unexpectedly for that. The first five patients whom I tested in this new way proved to have absolutely rigid stapes. The probe would not budge them. I scheduled them for subsequent Lempert fenestrations.

Then in came a young man who changed not only my life but the lives of millions of the hard of hearing throughout the world. We will call him Edward Lawrence. His story was typical of the victim of otosclerosis. All through his twenties his hearing had been slowly declining. Now he was in his early forties, and the handicap was becoming a serious problem both in his work and in his social life. Mr. Lawrence was a chemical engineer. To perform competently in his profession, it was absolutely essential that he hear precisely what was being said at meetings, in noisy factories, in all kinds of situations. Guessing at what is being said in a conference on technical matters is a risky business at best, and Mr. Lawrence, a highly intelligent man, was well aware of the dangers to his career and to the men he worked with if he should make some foolish mistake as a result of misunderstanding, or rather mishearing, some vital point. He was by now desperately worried about his career, about his future, and he was determined to do something about it. In fact, he already had. He had been to specialists in Chicago and Baltimore. Both had told him that he had otosclerosis and advised a Lempert fenestration. A friend on whom I had performed a successful fenestration had suggested that he consult me before agreeing to the operation. It was typical of his thoroughness that he had brought with him the audiograms and reports of the other doctors, but I had my own audiologist run him through the tests again just to be sure.

Afterwards he came into my consulting room and we got down to cases. I raised my voice. The tests, I told him, confirmed the findings of the men he had already seen. He probably had a progressive overgrowth of bone that was gradually freezing the footplate of the stapes and preventing vibrations from reaching the inner ear. The procedure that had restored hearing in his friend might also help him.

"So let's get on with it, doctor," he said at once.

I raised my hand. "Not so fast, Mr. Lawrence. In the first place, I have to be sure you understand that fenestration is not always successful, and it never restores hearing to completely normal levels." I went on, describing the risks involved, the possibility that the operation would injure the auditory nerve, irremediably causing a worsening of the hearing in that ear, and the other unpleasant facts of medical life in this uncertain world of ours. I always take my patients completely into my confidence in this way, because, after all, the decision is not mine to make but theirs, and they can make it intelligently only if they know all the facts, favorable and unfavorable, certain and uncertain.

Then I explained my idea about the preliminary diagnostic

operation. He was an engineer, and so I went into precise detail, describing what we know about the physics and the physiology of hearing. I told him why it was desirable to know whether or not his stapes was still mobile, because if it were, that knowledge would preclude subjecting him needlessly to the fenestration operation.

He nodded. Without a moment's hesitation he elected to have me perform the diagnostic operation. I scheduled it for the next day.

When he was wheeled into the operating room at Mount Sinai he was drowsy from the medication I had ordered but still businesslike and cheerful. The nurse handed me my funnel-shaped ear speculum and a hypodermic syringe containing Novocain.

"Now, you're going to feel a little pin prick in the ear," I said loudly. "That's all the pain you'll feel, because this is the local anesthetic that I'm going to inject. The rest of it won't take very long—maybe ten or fifteen minutes at most."

"Take your time, doc," he answered cheerily from beneath the surgical drapes covering his head. I turned on my head lamp and began to inject the anesthetic at three points deep in the ear canal. Then, using a surgical separator, I began to peel the skin of the canal down to the level of the eardrum. Once this was done, I could fold half of the drum forward like an apron, exposing the contents of the middle ear that lay beneath the drum. Unlike some patients, the anatomy of Mr. Lawrence's middle ear was such that I could plainly see the stapes in the binocular magnifying loupes that I was wearing.

"May I have the probe, please?" I asked my nurse.

I placed the needle-sharp tip of the probe against the head of the stapes and exerted a rapid, pulsating pressure on it in the direction it would normally move if it were not fixed in place by disease.

It seemed to me that perhaps it moved. What a disappointment! I had so wanted to help this man, but if the stapes was mobile, it was a virtual certainty that he would not benefit from fenestration. I was so absorbed in my unhappy thoughts that for a moment I did not notice that there was now a little bleeding in the middle ear.

"Suction, please," I said quietly.

"Dr. Rosen!" Mr. Lawrence suddenly said. "I can hear you! I can hear everything now, things I haven't heard for so many years."

"What?" I asked stupidly.

"Honest, doc. I heard you just as plain as anything," he said urgently. "Listen. I can prove it to you. Just a second ago I heard somebody drop something made of metal. It was outside of this room somewhere."

Thinking about it for a moment, I realized that he was right. I too had heard some nurse drop an instrument into an operating room pail. It was the kind of familiar sound that, during the intense concentration of surgery, one learns to ignore, lest he be distracted from the exacting work he is doing. But I suddenly realized that the sound had come from far down the corridor in another operating room. It had passed through two heavy doors to reach this room, and it was really quite faint.

"Yes," I whispered. "You're right. I heard it too. Can you hear me now, Mr. Lawrence?"

"Sure can," he said exultantly. The satisfaction in his voice was immense, but I had asked many patients that question and long since learned never to rely on the answer. It's too obvious; the patient has too powerful a need to have his hopes fulfilled and so he often guesses correctly what question is being asked.

"Do you like your eggs scrambled or fried?" I whispered very softly.

"Oh, I prefer them scrambled," the engineer replied at once.

I was thunderstruck. Looking up at the nurse, I saw her experienced eyes brimming with tears. We had worked together many times through many laborious hours of fenestration surgery to achieve a less dramatic result, and here was a patient who, after a simple operation lasting only a few minutes, could hear the merest whisper. But it was no time for exultation; it was a time for cool thinking, and first of all, of thinking about the patient.

I patted him on his draped shoulder, and said as calmly as possible: "Well, I guess that's enough of that for today. We'll send you off to bed now, and I'll see you in the morning and we'll talk about this whole matter then, okay?"

"Anything you say, doc," he said, "but I can hear! I can hear!"

# Of Politics and Medicine

---

I knew that a long, tedious investigation lay ahead of me, but the circumstances were such that I had plenty of time to pursue it. Of course, I had the motive to do so, born of my years of training in my specialty and my long habit of curiosity.

The time was created, ironically, by what had happened to Helen and me as a result of our interest in political and social questions. During the war it had been possible to be active in liberal and even in radical causes without incurring the wrath of the medical establishment. It was a war against fascism, after all, and so to be against fascism was now suddenly fairly respectable. The pressures of wartime practice were fierce, but even so I found time to participate with Helen, particularly in the Independent Citizens Committee of the Arts, Sciences, and Professions. The ICCASP, usually called simply "the ASP," was created in the early 1940's to muster support for Franklin Roosevelt's fourth-term presidential candidacy. Thousands of the country's most renowned actors, writers, artists, scientists, and other professionals took part in it. We were brought into it by Fredric March and his wife, Florence Eldridge, who were fellow parents at the Dalton School. They had a country place near ours and their children were about the same ages as ours.

Helen had been driving an ambulance for the American Women's Voluntary Services during the war, but she was no longer needed. She welcomed the opportunity to work in the ASP. Its headquarters was in the Astor Hotel on Times Square. Around the corner Paul Robeson was playing *Othello*. He often dropped in to the ASP office because he was very active in the organization. Helen invited him to our house for dinner, and we soon became fast friends. I felt as if I had always known him, because of something that had happened when I was a college student.

I was a great sports fan then, and still am. One of the things I liked to do was to get at least a glimpse of the players before the game, then watch the game, then see if I couldn't catch sight of a particular player afterwards. In that way I felt that I knew much more about some athlete whose performance had caught my eye. It was a form of hero-worship, perhaps. I was certainly no star athlete. I was too short and too skinny.

One day Syracuse played against Rutgers University. The unquestioned star of the game was the lone black player on the Rutgers team, left end Paul Robeson. He was a superb performer and an All-American in 1918. After the game was over, I lingered near the entrance to the stadium gymnasium to watch the players as they left. The Syracuse team, beaten but perfectly cheerful about it, emerged from the gym. A few minutes later the Rutgers team appeared. The boys laughed, yelled, joked. They formed little groups in the corridor, linked arms, and left. Soon everyone but Robeson had gone. Then he appeared. He walked alone down the long corridor toward the exit. Not a soul with him. He was completely abandoned by his teammates.

It was the first time that I really understood what it meant to be black. My heart went out to him. I wished I could put my arm around him and walk with him. I was unutterably sad. It tormented me for years. Here was a man who had everything—a brilliant student, a Phi Beta Kappa, a great athlete—yet his teammates walked out on him to their parties and their co-eds without a glance backward.

When we got to know him a quarter of a century later, I told him about this experience and how terrible I felt about it. We talked a lot about what life had done to us. It seemed to me that Paul and I had more in common than we had in differences, except that he was forever stamped by what this country does to people with black skin. Paul was as slow to acquire his political viewpoint as I. When he graduated from Columbia Law School, he took a job with a big New York firm. Soon he realized that he was being used as a "show Negro," a token of the firm's alleged liberalness. Actually, he was just a glorified office boy. In some way he had gotten to know Alexander Woollcott, the brilliant critic and essayist. Woollcott had heard Paul sing spirituals and arranged a concert for him at the Provincetown Playhouse. It was an instant success. Realizing that he could make his own way by his dramatic talents, Paul dropped the law and built a career as an actor and singer. Gradually, he turned more and more to the left in politics. He never forgot his origins. He never forgot what it was like to be poor, to be abandoned, to be rejected, and so he always sided with the poor.

Needless to say, our association with a black, no matter how brilliant he might be, no matter how famous, did not sit particularly well with my colleagues at the hospital. But we really didn't much care. We were too interested in what was going on in the world, in the peace that was looming closer and closer, and in the postwar world. I have said that doctors tend to be rather naïve politically. Perhaps this was true of me too. After the war, we thought that the United States and the Soviet Union would remain allies. An era of peace and progress would ensue in which the two superpowers would cooperate to put an end to the gulf that separated the "have" from the "have-not" nations of the world. So we thought, but, as everyone knows, F.D.R. was hardly laid to rest before the Cold War began. Overnight Russia became "the enemy," and every political viewpoint left of center in this country was labeled "Communist." President Truman's policies created a deep split in the Democratic Party, with the result that some of its best men left. One of the most eminent was former Vice President Henry A. Wallace. He had been Truman's Secretary of Commerce. When Henry Wallace resigned and moved to South Salem, New York, Helen and I held a huge welcoming party for him. We already knew him well, because soon after the war ended he gravitated toward the group of New Yorkers who were concerned about what was happening, especially in foreign policy.

It was the end of an era, but the end was drawn out by the 1948 presidential campaign. Henry ran on the Progressive Party ticket. By then we knew him well and had become ardent supporters of his candidacy. Only when the campaign was over and the results were tallied did we realize how tiny a following a man like Henry Wallace could attract in this country. He got something over a million votes, doing only slightly better in absolute figures than Eugene V. Debs, the Socialist Party candidate in 1912!

It was a sign of the times. In the next years, the country moved rapidly to the right. Anti-Communist hysteria was the plaything of politicians of every stripe, from Joseph McCarthy to Hubert Humphrey. Liberals vied with reactionaries to show how fierce they were in their opposition to what they called "communism."

In our experience, an event that took place in 1949 signaled for any who cared to pay attention what lay ahead. The Civil

Rights Congress had scheduled an outdoor summer concert in Peekskill, New York, not far from our summer place. Paul Robeson was to sing. There were others whom we also knew who were participating because they believed, as we did, that the work of the CRC was important. At the time, the organization was mainly trying to raise funds for the defense of American Communists who had been indicted for "conspiracy to advocate" the overthrow of the federal government. We wanted to help, because we believed that the real threat to democracy then was in such efforts to suppress dissenting opinion, just as we think today that the "Chicago Seven," the Berrigans, and the Angela Davis conspiracy trials threaten everyone's freedom.

I believe that political parties should have an opportunity freely to get across their point of view to the people. Indicting the whole leadership of a party, no matter if it was an unpopular party, was not Helen's or my idea of how to preserve freedom—not just freedom for the Communists, but freedom for everybody. When one group gets it in the neck, the rest had better keep a sharp eye out for the next swing of the governmental ax.

Helen and I had no plan to attend the Robeson concert in Peekskill. I had been in an automobile accident and was in a heavy cast. Our son, John, was due home from camp. Paul called from Grand Central Station in New York. The American Legion, the Veterans of Foreign Wars, the Jewish War Veterans, and other right-wing groups, he had heard, were making trouble, threatening to break up the concert. They made good their threat. They stoned and overturned the cars of concertgoers, while the New York State troopers looked on approvingly. It was a police-assisted riot, not much different from the Chicago police riot of 1968 during the Democratic National Convention. There was no concert.

That night a member of the concert committee called us. He said that the riot had been planned to frighten people away, that it was a little Reichstag fire. Would we, he wanted to know, allow a protest rally to be held on our lawn the next day? Helen and I discussed it. If they had asked to use the place for something else, I don't know what I would have said, but I was good and mad. The very idea of men who are supposed to protect the weak and the helpless standing by while toughs attacked women and children enraged me.

"It's going to complicate our lives," I said, "but tell him they can hold the rally here."

In an hour the news was on the radio and the next day three thousand people swarmed onto our lawn, listened to the speakers, and voted by acclamation to hold the concert benefit the following week at a nearby fairgrounds.

I soon found out how naïve I had been when I had said that this might "complicate" our lives. The day after the rally my office was almost empty of patients. There was one phone call from a woman on whose son I had done a particularly delicate mastoid operation in the days before antibiotics, and the lad had been in desperate condition. It was nip and tuck to save his life, and I had stopped by at the hospital two and three times a day to be sure that he was all right, that the infection had really been controlled, that he was on the road to recovery. Of course, the woman couldn't say enough good things about me when her son finally returned home well and whole.

Now she phoned. She had heard on the radio about the rally at our home in Katonah.

"I had an appointment with you next week, Dr. Rosen," she said without preliminaries. "Cancel it. No money of mine is going to the Commies."

She hung up immediately, and that was just as well. A physician should be slow to reply in kind to a patient, but there are limits to what can be expected of anyone.

In the next weeks my office staff had many opportunities

to practice the soft answer that turneth away wrath, but with very limited success. My practice dwindled to almost nothing. At least one trustee at Mount Sinai Hospital said, according to a trustee who told me about it secretly, that "any man who had been for Henry Wallace and who had been at Peekskill" (I hadn't) must be a Communist and that Mount Sinai should get rid of him.

If this ever came formally before the board of trustees, however, those gentlemen must have had cooler heads. Nothing happened. I continued as a member of the hospital staff. My wealthier patients tended to disappear, but poor people continued to come—and people who didn't know me and so didn't know they were entrusting their bodies, or at least their ears and their immortal souls, to a dangerous, atheistic Bolshevist.

Some of the physicians who had regularly referred cases to me stopped. Others stubbornly continued to send me patients whom they felt needed my special skills. Their confidence in my abilities as a surgeon and their insistence on thinking first of their patients' interests overcame their political misgivings or opposition. Some of them at that time of extreme hysteria must have been convinced that Helen and I were dangerous Reds. Others who knew better kept right on knowing better, although they must also have known that it would do them no great good in professional circles to persist in referring patients to me. These men kept alive my faith in the fundamental decency of some part of any group of individuals, even physicians. There are always a few who on principle—whether the principle be philosophical or otological—will not be stampeded into betraying their own best judgment and their own standards of what is decent and what is obscene. I am not going to name them. The Cold War is still with us late and soon, and who knows what indignities my grateful mention of their names might later visit upon them. They know who they are and they ought to know that they represent the finest traditions of the profession.

At a time like that you find out who your friends really are. A good many of them had long since come to regard our political tendencies as just an unfortunate aberration that had to be tolerated out of loyalty and love. To them, we were friends who had suddenly developed some particularly unpleasant deformity, but who were still the same people they had always loved, and they were damned if they were going to abandon us in our hour of need. Henry Wallace, whose friendship abided, was one of those who disagreed strongly with us. He thought we were making a terrible mistake in thus exposing ourselves to public opprobrium.

"There are times when you plant and expect fruit," he said. "There are other times when you plant a seed, and it just will not sprout, just *will not grow*."

I think that was the closest he could come to expressing his concern. Henry was a kindly person, but he was not a warm man. He was an undemonstrative, very ungraceful, profoundly lonely man. It was hard to answer him, but it would have been an insult to a man of such integrity and decency not to tell him how we felt.

"I realize that, Henry," I said, "but we feel we have to do what we have to do. I'm very mindful of what you say, and we are not doing this out of some stiff-necked pride or something. Sometimes seeds remain dormant for a long time. At least if they are planted, they have a chance sometime to come to life."

Another close friend during those difficult times was Dashiell Hammett. He had no problem in understanding our position because, if anything, he was even more staunch in his determination to stand up for his political views. Rather than give a New York official the names of individuals who had posted bail for Communists and other left-wing dissenters, Dash served six months in prison. When he was released, he came to live in a little cottage on our place. We grew to delight in his lean, laconic wit and to relish his sardonic outlook on life. He absolutely refused to take seriously those betrayals by friends that were routine in a time when one intellectual after another was summoned to testify before the House Committee on Un-American Activities. One of these was a motion picture producer and writer who was later brought by our house in Katonah when he was the guest of a neighbor. The man had testified about many of his old friends and acquaintances—to their extreme detriment, of course, although the worst he had really been able to say was that maybe they had supported Communist or left-wing causes at some time or other in the past. When Helen learned who he was, she peremptorily asked him to leave. After one look at Helen, he prudently decided to depart, accompanied by his host.

Dash laughed.

"You're nuts, Helen," he said. "People are what they are. Why didn't you invite him in and give him a drink?"

Helen was outraged at such an idea.

Fresh from prison because he would not turn over the names of persons whom he did not even know, Dash just shrugged his shoulders.

"Aw, you take things too seriously, Helen," he said.

Still, I agree with Helen. To betray one of the most precious things of life, the trust and friendship of others—such an act is unforgivable.

During that Cold War period in the early 1950's, one never knew what would happen next, who would prove to be friend, who would betray. To join in this obscene orgy of betrayal would have been to sink to a level lower than my worst detractors. I believe in loyalty, loyalty to one's principles, to the best traditions of one's country.

I remember the Sunday that President Truman authorized the sending of American troops under General MacArthur into Korea in force. He called it a "police action," but it was war, regardless of the legalistic niceties. A group of us were sitting on our porch. There were Clifford Odets, the playwright; Gregory Zilboorg, the psychoanalyst; Jack McManus, the editor; Henry Wallace; and no doubt some others. Many of us felt that it was shocking that the President had in effect declared war without congressional approval, without consultation. Some of us, including myself, thought that the Korean war might well have been provoked by some scheme of Mr. Truman's emissary to South Korea, John Foster Dulles, later Secretary of State under President Eisenhower.

No matter. The point is that, of all of us, Henry was very upset in a different way. He detested Harry Truman, but it was clear that he was in deep conflict. Someone suggested that perhaps what we were watching was another episode in the general pattern of anti-Communist foreign adventures by America, the result of which seemed to be that small nations end up becoming client states of the United States.

"That's probably perfectly true," Henry said sadly, "but now that we are involved in actual war, I must support my country. Right or wrong I must support America."

He soon withdrew from the Progressive Party of which he had been the founder, and as time passed he dropped all political and social activity. Yet our friendship stood as fast as ever. He had done what he could do, and when he could do no more, he simply ceased and went back to his first love—the cultivation of plants and animals.

Perhaps all this is of such great importance to me because of my desperately poor origins, the son of an incompetent peddler of crockery, and the product, in the last analysis, of my mother's, my sister's, and my brothers' steady encouragement and support, both emotional and financial.

During that frenzied Cold War period it seemed that any man might turn on another. If this happened, it meant that we would once more find ourselves thrown back on very meager resources in a hostile world. We had a lovely summer home, a daughter in college and a son just finishing preparatory school, and we had our political and social ideals. For the sake of political principle or religious belief the most awful crimes have been committed throughout history by supposedly respectable men. We had reason to feel gravely threatened with the loss of all that we had achieved over the years.

Ironically, the very threat was also a challenge. My practice had faded away, but Mr. Lawrence had presented me with an opportunity that a more respectable, and hence far busier surgeon, might have overlooked. I had plenty of time to pursue and perfect.

# Of the Living and the Dead

Chance favors the prepared mind. When, in the 1930's, Alexander Fleming was working with the *Staphylococcus aureus* microbe, he found one of his cultures contaminated by a mold. It had undoubtedly happened before to investigators who must have promptly discarded the culture. But Dr. Fleming noticed that around each tiny colony of the mold called *Penicillium*, there was a "demilitarized zone." Nothing grew there. The mold produced something that inhibited the growth of the "staph." After much painstaking research, that something was isolated and identified as penicillin.

Now, except perhaps to the hard of hearing, the discovery of stapes mobilization is not in the same class with the discovery of penicillin. The point here is only that, odd though it may seem, most of my colleagues have told me that they would almost certainly have ignored what happened to Mr. Lawrence as "just a fluke." This has always seemed incredible to me. How could anyone disregard so dramatic a development? I felt like a man who has just won the sweepstakes—happy and incredulous, because although we know that *someone* always wins, we figure it's never going to be us. We are not really prepared, psychologically, for lightning to strike.

What makes the mind "prepared" for the completely novel, the wholly unexpected? When I was a child, I used to have a recurrent dream. I would be walking along a country road. As I looked down at the dirt road, I would just be able to make out the glinting edge of what looked like a coin. I would kick away the dirt and lo! there would be a whole nickel, and I would say to my dreaming self, "My goodness, how great! how wonderful!" Then I would begin kicking all around that first nickel. Another and another and another would appear in the dusty road, until suddenly I found myself in a pit filled with nickels. In the dream I would then run home, get a wheelbarrow and shovel, and load up the nickels. Five cents was a fabulous treasure to a poor little boy.

The dream seems very meaningful. It is vital to hold on to the dreams and visions of childhood. Those are the ones that are rich and that point you in the right direction. When Mr. Lawrence suddenly heard clearly again, it was as if I had once more seen the glint of that first nickel. Nothing could stop me from looking further.

He had been operated on late in the afternoon. I left the hospital bursting with tension. The conviction filled me that my life had reached an important turning point. From now on, nothing would be the same. As I walked home through the city, I felt that I had to keep moving, had to hurry. I was like a nervous bridegroom who rushes to his wedding but has forgotten to tie his tie!

Helen was home. In a rush of words, I told her what had happened.

"Oh, Sam!" she exclaimed. "That's absolutely marvelous."

"Well, I don't know," I said. "It depends."

"On what, Sam?" she asked.

"Maybe it was just an accident. Maybe I won't be able to repeat it and get the same results. Maybe it wasn't anything I did at all but just some kind of fluke."

"You'll know the answer to that soon enough, won't you?" she said. "You'll try it on new cases, and then you'll know."

"I can't," I told her. "Too risky, especially since I'm not absolutely sure of what I did to bring this about. I was just checking the man to be sure a 'Lempert' would work on him, and now look at him: he can hear normally, and I'm not sure I know how I did it.

"Maybe it will turn out to be just a ten-day or a ninety-day wonder, and then he will go back to the same condition he had before. Maybe—God, I hope not!—maybe I restored his hearing but caused some damage to the nerve of hearing that won't appear until later."

Helen, who had worked long and often with me on research that interested both of us, understood perfectly. She prepared supper quietly, leaving me to my thoughts. Helen is a great cook. No doubt dinner was delicious, but that night I ate mechanically, paying not the least attention to anything around me. I went over the entire operation in my mind, hoping to think of something that I had not yet recalled. Each time I got to the point where my explorer was on the man's stapes and I was exerting a gentle, rhythmic pressure. At that moment he was saying nothing, but seconds later he was crying: "I can hear!" I was firmly convinced that this sequence of events plainly pointed to but one conclusion: that Mr. Lawrence's stapes had not been firmly embedded in the otosclerotic growth and that, consequently, I had loosened it from its bonds.

To be useful to science, an experiment has to be replicable, so that others can try it out independently of the original experimenter. Repeating an experiment this way is the standard method by which scientists validate a new discovery. And since this "experiment" also held the potential of being a major new procedure in ear surgery, there could be no room for doubt. Furthermore, I knew there was another complication: Human anatomy is incredibly varied, and the middle ear is such a tiny space that the least variation from one patient's ear to another might pose insuperable problems. Moreover, there were other risks to which patients must not be exposed: The instrument I had used was designed only for the purpose of palpating the stapes, that is, of feeling the mobility or immobility of the tiny bone. If I tried experimenting on living patients, I might easily blunder and injure the facial nerve, causing paralysis of one side of the face.

Sleep was impossible that night, so I got out my microscope and looked at slides through it, just to keep myself occupied. Some people have dogs or cats for pets. Mine is a beautiful old Zeiss microscope used sometimes for research, other times just to explore the amazing microscopic world that is as much around us as are the stars.

By morning, I had worked it out. I had a good idea of what the problems were and a clear-cut program for finding the answers to them.

My first step along that torturous road was to call Dr. Leo Stern, my dentist and friend. Lying awake, I had been wondering where on earth I could get instruments that would enable me to reach the stapes and apply pressure in various ways and directions to it. In my mind's eye, I saw Leo's round white tray. On it was an array of delicate instruments of all shapes and sizes, perfect for working in confined spaces.

Leo told me that S. S. White on 42nd Street was the place to get instruments of that kind. I wanted to rush off there at once, but patients were already gathering in the waiting room of my office. Some had otosclerosis. "If mobilization worked for Lawrence, then why not for this woman?" I kept thinking. Why not? No. It was a wholly untested procedure. To attempt it on a living patient would have been to violate the physician's most fundamental code of conduct: *Primum non nocere,* first do no harm.

When finally my office hours were over, I went to the hospital to see my "miracle" patient. He did not look especially happy. His hearing had dropped back. My heart sank. I removed the packing in the ear and whispered: "How do you like your steaks cooked, Mr. Lawrence?"

He grinned ecstatically.

"Rare, Dr. Rosen! Rare. Were you whispering, really whispering?"

"As softly as I do to my wife," said I, delightedly.

I replaced the packing with fresh cotton—nothing more was needed. Then I sat down on the edge of the bed and looked at my forty-year-old "wunderkind" soberly, right in the eye.

"Now, Mr. Lawrence," I said. "We have a measure of good fortune, you and I, and I think I understand what has happened. In testing the mobility of your stapes, I freed it, so now you can hear quite normally in that ear—*for the time being. For the time being.* Mr. Lawrence, it would be hard to overemphasize that. Your hearing in that ear will probably drop back below where it was, at least for a time because of swelling of the tissues. It may even get worse and stay that way until we do the Lempert's on it."

"You mean you're going to do the fenestration?" he asked incredulously. He was a highly intelligent patient. "I don't need it."

"Of course you don't," I agreed. "Not now, anyway. But what I want to be sure we both understand is that this may not last. I feel quite certain that no permanent harm has been done, but I have no way of knowing whether the good that has been done is temporary or permanent.

"Now, what is terribly important to me, and to a lot of other people who may benefit by this—what is absolutely crucial is that you keep in touch with me. I *have* to know exactly what happens to you, and unfortunately, you live in the Midwest, and, well, frankly, Mr. Lawrence, I am extremely anxious to have your assurance that you will keep in close touch with me at all times for the next few months and then will come back for further testing of that ear."

It was a stroke of real luck that Mr. Lawrence was a highly trained, professional man. He understood my problem instantly and was good enough to assure me that he would faithfully call in and report on his status at regular intervals.

"Of course I will," he said, and added matter-of-factly as an afterthought: "It's obviously in my interest to follow through on this too, doctor."

Vastly relieved, I signed his hospital discharge. In the days and weeks that followed, I was haunted by an utterly unreasonable sense of abandonment. After all, the man had his work to do, but if I could have had my way, I would have kept him locked up in our guest room until I could finish the work that I knew I had to do.

Leaving the hospital, I rushed down to 42nd Street to the S. S. White showroom. What an assortment of instruments there were: literally hundreds, each varying ever so slightly from another in curve, thickness, length. Some were shaped for use on the right side; some for the left; some were sharp, some needle-like; some were blunt, some pointed; some had cutting edges; some were spoon-shaped; some were like tiny chisels. I felt like a kid in a toy store—and acted accordingly. Instead of buying a few of the most likely-looking instruments, I blew three or four hundred dollars. I have often wondered since what the delighted salesman thought of me. He couldn't have been too dissatisfied, since I paid immediately and rushed off with my treasure. It would have made more sense to buy six or seven at a time and then to go back for more, but that was not my mood. This might be the only time and place to get them. I had to have every possible instrument, so that if one would not do the job, I could try another.

I took them straight home. No one was in. I was glad of that, because I wanted to think about the instruments without distraction. I spread them out on my desk and looked at them lovingly, trying to visualize just where and how I might use each one in the middle ear. This was the beginning of a long love affair with my instruments. I would take them off to where I could be alone with them—to the garage in the country, to my bedroom in the city—and I would look at them, feel them, work the business end of an instrument under my thumbnail to feel how it penetrated, how it felt when pressure was exerted on it. I would study the instrument's shape and curve, examine the cutting edge, get the feel of the instrument so as to combine that with my intimate knowledge of middle-ear anatomy and form an idea of precisely how each one might be used in stapes mobilization. Sometimes I would use a thick-skinned apple or orange for practice. At other times I would just fondle the instrument, running my finger lightly over its working surfaces, thinking about it, touching it, feeling it, seeing what it felt like on my skin. I got in the habit of carrying one or two in my jacket pocket. Even at parties I would sit talking to someone while all the time surreptitiously hefting one of those instruments, pressing it against my skin or nail or manipulating it. It must have been an odd sight for visitors, Dr. Rosen twiddling not his thumbs but his pet instruments.

Devising new instruments was only part of the problem. Describing his technique for operating on the facial nerve, Sir Charles Ballance wrote: " . . . the surgeon learned in anatomy, and with the knowledge learned in the deadhouse, may safely traverse the perilous narrow ocean . . ." I was learned in the anatomy of the middle ear, but the knowledge had to be applied. It occurred to me that Lempert somehow always had cadavers available for the students who came to New York to take his course in fenestration surgery. Nobody knew where he got them, and Lempert never volunteered the information. I soon learned why he was so circumspect about this one subject, but meanwhile, I was at a loss to solve my own problem—Mount Sinai, then not a teaching hospital, could not be a source of cadavers—and I knew there would be no point in asking Lempert. . . . But the deadhouse. I recalled the diener at Syracuse Medical School. A diener's job is to prepare the cadavers, house them in a cold room, bring them up to the gross anatomy laboratory for the use of students, dispose of parts that have been dissected and studied, and finally to remove the flesh by boiling the cadaver in some corrosive liquid so that students would have a complete skeleton for use in studying osteology. (Before going on, let me say that much of what follows in this chapter is not exactly light reading. The fastidious reader may prefer to skip to the next chapter.)

The diener (a German word for "servant") at Syracuse was in my student days a short, soft-spoken man in his middle forties. He said very little, but regarded us students with his dark brown eyes. He always wore a black rubber apron. Tony liked us, and we liked him—and for a special reason. If you lost a bone, you had to pay for it. Students soon learned to ask Tony if he could supply the missing part. The diener insisted on some plausible explanation for why the bone was missing, but we were quick to learn that this was only a formality and that he invariably managed to produce a replacement.

Once when I went down to the morgue to ask Tony to replace a bone, he was busy cutting off the head of a cadaver. It did not strike me as unusual at the time, but now it occurred to me that there had been absolutely no reason for Tony to be doing that, unless he was obliging some faculty member or a doctor in private practice. Was it possible that one or more of the dieners of the New York medical schools might be similarly obliging?

The day after I bought my treasure trove of instruments, I went and looked up the diener at a certain medical school. We will call it the Manhattan University School of Medicine and, without pretensions, its diener, Mr. Diener.

He was at his desk in the basement next to the huge doors of the refrigerated room where he kept his cadavers. When I began explaining my problem, Mr. Diener quickly interrupted me.

"Let's go in here to discuss this, doctor," he suggested. He opened the door to the refrigerated room and politely stepped back to let me go first.

Inside were at least fifty cadavers. The brightly lighted room was equipped with an overhead monorail along which rolled steel-gray trolleys; from these each cadaver was suspended by two curved pieces of metal hinged like ice tongs. The ends of the tongs had been inserted in the ear canals. It was a big-city set-up, coldly efficient compared to Tony's makeshift arrangements at Syracuse.

The diener closed the door behind us without a glance at the assembled company of naked men and women, and said: "All right, doctor. Nobody'll overhear us in here."

I hoped he was right.

"Well, you see it's like this, Mr. Diener," I said earnestly. "I'm developing a new ear operation and I desperately need heads for experimental purposes. What I need is a head with an intact ear on both sides."

Mr. Diener looked down at the glistening tile floor. The air in the room was so cold we could see the water vapor in our exhalations. We must have looked like a pair of demonic conspirators, standing there amid that congregation of deceased New Yorkers who had eyes to see and ears to hear but no breath of life.

"I've never done such a thing in my life," Mr. Diener said quietly. "If anyone found out, it would cost me my job. Maybe worse than that, Dr. Rosen, because this thing you're asking is absolutely illegal."

The only sound in the refrigerated room was the faint hum of the cooling machinery. The diener still had his hand on the door latch as if he were ready to make a quick escape from the room.

"Honest, Mr. Diener," I pleaded, "I'll be absolutely discreet. You can bank on that. Nobody but you and me will know anything about it. I've just *got* to have specimens to work on. I can't do this thing on a living patient until I know exactly what I'm doing. You understand how that is, don't you?

"Besides," I rushed on, "if it's illegal for you, just think of what might happen if anyone found out I was doing this. I could lose my license to practice. No, sir, you don't have to worry about *my* keeping my mouth shut."

But Mr. Diener was the soul of caution. "Where you gonna work on them, doctor?" he asked.

"In absolute secrecy," I assured him. "Nobody will see me."

"Well, I've never done this, Dr. Rosen," he said dubiously. He looked at the suspended rows of cadavers. "Ear canals have to be intact too?"

"No. Only the middle ear," I said. "Any of these would do very well, provided there's been no damage to the middle ear. How far do those things go into the ear canal?"

"Just a couple of centimeters."

"Then you'll do it?" I asked eagerly. "I'll be glad to pay you whatever you think right for each head."

The diener looked around the room, as though he were in silent consultation with his charges.

"Well, I'll have to think about it, Dr. Rosen," he said. "Tell you what. You call me tomorrow, and I'll let you know."

"I'd rather not phone you," I said. "Suppose I drop in on you about four thirty tomorrow?"

"All right," he said.

The next day we talked some more. Finally the diener said: "Come back here tomorrow night about nine o'clock."

When I arrived the following evening he nodded quickly and disappeared into the cold room, returning with something wrapped in white oilcloth. He placed this in a cardboard carton and tied it with a cord.

"Seventy-five dollars, please." I paid him in cash and walked out, carrying the box as carefully as if it contained a million dollars. I placed the box in the trunk of my car and drove off, making a special effort to pay attention to the traffic, pedestrians, traffic lights. This was no time to get into trouble. I was as elated as a child with a new toy. Beside me on the seat were those precious, sharp, glinting pieces of steel with which it would surely be possible to enter the middle ear and manipulate that little rice-grain-sized bone in the ear. In the trunk I had the other essential for progress. Where to keep it?

Even assuming that Helen would have let me keep it there, the refrigerator at home would not hold it. The autopsy room at my hospital had a kind of anteroom, the left wall of which contained twenty stretchers in refrigerated racks that rolled silently out on bearings, like oversized filing cabinet drawers. The highest drawers were rarely used. Here was a safe place to hide my purchase.

"I'll be working on this nights," I explained to the Mount Sinai diener. If he was scandalized he showed no sign of it. I gave him five dollars. "Let's just keep it quiet, shall we?"

The next evening, after a quick supper, I gathered up my instruments, my magnifying loupes (fitted to spectacle frames so that I could look into the ear at 2 times magnification), and my headlight, a device that looks much like a miner's headlamp.

In the autopsy room I opened the box. Within the folds of oilcloth was the ravaged countenance of a man of about fifty. He had a few days' growth of beard. His cheeks were sunken from the effects of years of alcoholism. His nose was long and aquiline, his mouth small and almost fretful, and he seemed to have very large external ears. He had no doubt been a derelict—a term often used today with derision and contempt, but one that always fills me with sorrow and shame. Most of those whose bodies are turned over for research or education in this country are the refuse of society, the wrecks of what were once smiling children, gentle lovers, and tender mothers and fathers. They are mute witnesses to society's ultimate abandonment, its final act of alienation. No wonder we fear the cadaver, for it is a symbol of all that we most dread: of being unwanted, unwept in the final hours of life.

At least my unwanted man would have a last opportunity to make a great gift, to me and through me to the human race. The autopsy room at Mount Sinai that night was filled with the hope that this silent outcast might prove to be a friend who could do something no other had the power to do: reveal the secrets of what had happened to Mr. Lawrence and show me how it could be done again and again. Of one thing I was sure. This man was neither judge nor prosecutor. He sat on no boards of trustees or congressional committees. He would not judge, but the gift of his body would soon reveal whether my highest hopes had any substance in the cold clay of mortal tissue.

# Of Adventure by Night

---

I placed the head on one of the autopsy tables in the same position that the head of a living patient would normally be during an operation on the middle ear, adjusted my headlight, put on the loupe, and inserted the funnel-shaped speculum. These accustomed acts drove all thoughts from my mind except those that had to do with the task immediately at hand. With a scalpel, I incised the skin inside the ear canal, drawing an incision from what would be about twelve o'clock to six o'clock on a watch face. This makes it possible to fold back the eardrum without disturbing the ossicles. With a curette, an instrument whose cutting edge is cup-shaped, one then carves away just enough bone in the forward part of the canal to expose the incus and stapes.

It was thrilling. Here was the minuscule stage on which a drama affecting millions would be acted out. There lay the target: the neck of the stapes, where the two tiny arms of bone that arise from the footplate join together and articulate with the incus. The first problem was to devise an instrument that would reach over the incus and contact the stapes neck so that backward pressure could be safely exerted on it, without touching any of the other delicate parts of the middle ear. If the stapes could be moved backward by pressure at this point, its ligament and muscle would then pull it back to normal position; but if too much pressure were applied, there was the possibility of fracturing the stapes.

Night after night I spent hours in the Mount Sinai autopsy room, trying different instruments, selecting five or six that seemed most readily modifiable to perform exactly as required. With the help of the hospital's chief engineer, I finally got what I thought would be the proper curve in the tip of one instrument. That night I tried it again on the same ear, but to my disappointment I found I had made the curve too great; yet when the curve was straightened somewhat, it would not reach the stapes neck.

It was discouraging. My skills with a lathe and grinding tools were practically nonexistent, and the hospital's machinists, though friendly and obliging, perhaps did not quite understand what I wanted. Besides, they had other things to do than cater to a fussy surgeon who was constantly pestering them about his damned instruments. Again dentistry came to the rescue. My friend Leo Stern suggested that I try instrument makers he knew. They were a couple named Grafrath who had a workshop on the fourth floor of a crumbling brick loft building in the Hell's Kitchen section of Manhattan, just west of the theatrical district. They worked all day at grinding wheels driven by belts powered by an electric motor. The place was full of wheels, magnifying glasses, hundreds of instruments in various stages of completion, emery dust, steel dust, gleaming bars of different steel alloys. I had brought the instrument that I could not shape correctly and explained my problem in words and by drawing crude sketches of what shape was needed.

Mr. Grafrath nodded: "Can do that, all right."

I was fidgety. "Can you perhaps do it while I wait?" I asked hopefully.

"Well, not a good idea, doctor," he said. "You're nervous. You make me nervous. I wouldn't use that thing, anyway." He pointed rather disdainfully at my much-tortured S. S. White instrument.

"I tell you what: you leave everything here and come back tomorrow. I got other orders to do, but I can tell you really need this right away—not like some of them, ask you to do it right away, quick! and then don't come back for a week, maybe. I tell you what. I will make two for you, not quite the same. Then you tell me which one works best."

Mr. Grafrath was a genius. One of the two, which he made from new steel, was perfect. With it I could manipulate the stapes just as I wanted to, and with a feeling of complete security about precisely the amount of pressure I was applying. The Grafraths made me half a dozen. I had to be sure of having enough on hand. Everything seemed so chancy. It was as if I had to guard against any unlucky break interfering with my reaching my objective.

It was hard to stay away from the Grafraths' little shop. It was in a loft building near the Hudson River, up three flights of rickety stairs. One had to push a button downstairs and wait for Fred Grafrath or his wife to buzz the latch to let you in. Upstairs the door to their shop was always locked. When you rang, Fred Grafrath would open it as far as a chain inside allowed and peer out at the caller. When he recognized you, he would close the door, release the chain, let you in quickly, and then shut, lock, and chain the door again.

I got used to this soon enough, and asked no questions. But I was curious about Fred and his work, and finally felt it would be all right to venture a different question:

"Don't you get sick of doing this day after day all these years?" I asked.

"Well, Dr. Rosen," the little man said confidentially, "I just love steel. I love the feel of it. I love the smell of it. I love the sound of it on a dry stone or a wet stone. I can tell just what's happening by the sound as I put pressure on it or ease up.

"And I like to see that instrument starting out as just a rough piece of steel and gradually I shape it into something and then I smooth it and polish it and taper it and put the point on it, or the knife edge, or the chisel edge, or whatever is wanted."

It was no problem at all for me to recognize in Fred Grafrath a kindred spirit. If he had asked me the same question about my work, I would have answered in very much the same way. The satisfaction was *in* the work itself, in the skillful use of your hands, your muscles, your body, in being able to use your nervous and muscular mechanism so precisely in response to what your mind had decided was needed in a particular instance.

I used to marvel at Fred's hands. They looked as if particles of steel had become permanently embedded in his thick fingers and blunt, scarified nails. Yet they were beautiful hands; they had so much feel in them. You could sense the pleasure he experienced when he would pick up an instrument to show me. He held the piece of shining stainless steel lovingly, turning it gently in the light and waiting for me to admire it.

It was a companionable thing to talk with Fred, but Mrs. Grafrath, who kept the firm's books of account, was all business.

"We're awfully glad to have you come up and see us, Dr. Rosen," she said one day. "Every time Fred says to me, he says: 'You know that Dr. Rosen, I like to talk to him. He always listens to what I have to say.'"

Naturally, I was very flattered that Fred thought so highly of me, but Mrs. Grafrath had business in mind: "You know, when you come he don't get much work done, so maybe you shouldn't be such a good listener?" She said this with a smile and raised her voice enough so that Fred could hear her over the sound of the whirring wheels, so I don't really think she meant it seriously.

The Grafraths made about a dozen other special instruments for me: a flat, smooth, spatulalike one to permit pushing away the drum without injuring it; two or three with needle points for separating adhesions and for teasing bits of bone into a position from which they could be picked out of the middle ear with tiny surgical forceps; and a new set of curettes. The conventional curettes, delicate as they were, were too crude for this work. There had to be several different ones, because a curette that was right for one cadaver would prove to be too large or too small in another, or it would be curved in the wrong way for some other task.

Now things began to go well. If a large curette was needed, it was within reach; if a small one, it was there. There was no longer any danger of blundering into the delicate structures of the middle ear by accident. Working within a space smaller than the length and diameter of the eraser on a pencil, I could do anything I pleased. There were refinements to be carried out, of course. Almost every day the Grafraths cheerfully undertook to reshape this instrument just the least bit this way, and this other one a hair that way, and make this one a little sharper, that one blunter, or thinner, or thicker.

During all this time I had been very cautious in my work with my one cadaver head. I had not touched the other ear at all, and had been extremely careful not to apply very much force to the stapes in the ear I had opened. The bone looked so tiny and fragile, and even though it was mobile, it seemed to be so easy to fracture. How strong was it? I decided to find out. I extracted it and took it home. The next day I toured the drugstores near my home and near the hospital, looking for a set of the old-fashioned brass weights pharmacists used to use when they actually compounded prescriptions for doctors, instead of dispensing them from bottles of tablets and capsules supplied by our affluent pharmaceutical industry. The weights were gone, most of them sold to antique dealers. But luck was with me. A druggist who ran a small, dingy store on First Avenue produced a box of weights.

"Here you are, doctor," he said. "What you want them for?"

"I want to test the breaking strength of a certain bone in the body," I explained.

"Help yourself," he said. "Don't use 'em any more. Times've changed."

"I'll leave a deposit," I suggested.

"Nope," he said, ushering me out. "Don't need 'em. Glad to be of help in your research, doctor."

Trotting home with the box tucked under my arm, I planned my test. With Duco cement, I fixed the extracted stapes to a piece of lucite clamped in a vise, took a piece of wire —.0004 tantalum or steel—and wound it around the neck of the 8-ounce weight and then adjusted my loupes so that I could wind the wire around the neck of the stapes. Then I let the wire slide through my fingers until it became taut. There hung the heavy weight suspended by the minuscule bone. It held. It looked like a fly holding up an elephant!

Crude as this test was, it was now clear that nature, as if anticipating my intentions, had made the tiny bone far stronger than normal use required. One could apply far more force to it, especially at the neck, than would be needed to mobilize it.

Now to concentrate on the main task: practicing the procedure on as many different cadavers as could be somehow acquired. I was a very experienced ear surgeon, but I was a novice at this new operation, and I knew it. It was absolutely essential to repeat this procedure over and over again, deliberately to study the ways in which one could make blunders that, in the living, would have had disastrous consequences—perhaps total loss of hearing in the operated ear. And there was also that factor that all experienced surgeons are aware of: anatomical variation. To a palm reader, the minute differences in fingerprints don't matter. To a detective they make all the difference. The parts of the human body are not identical like those of an automobile. Every surgeon knows this but, as I have said, to those who operate in large body cavities, the variations are less critical than they are for the ear surgeon. The least difference in the location of a nerve, muscle, tendon, or bone in so restricted a space can spell the difference between success and disaster. So it was a problem of obtaining as many cadavers on which to work as possible, both for acquiring skill and for perfecting minor but critical variants on my set of instruments so as to have a suitable instrument available in every case, regardless of anatomical variations.

One must also become familiar with the infinite variations one is going to encounter; differences in size and strength of the stapes, differences in position of the ossicles, of the footplate, of the size of everything. When I went to Indonesia to teach, I discovered that the Indonesians have extremely small ear canals, so that it is very difficult to perform stapes mobilizations on them without extensive curettage of the canal walls. There are many other difficulties that anatomical idiosyncrasies present to the surgeon: the footplate may be located down in a deep recess at the entrance to the inner ear, making it difficult to see and to reach. The stapes varies from long and thin to short and thin to long and heavy, to short and heavy, and so on.

Intentionally attempting to mobilize the stapes of a living patient would have to wait until my hand had acquired the feel of doing it on many, many cadavers, and even on monkeys, whose ears are so delicate that, if you can mobilize the rhesus monkey stapes without injury to it or to the ear, you can surely have confidence in your ability to do so in the most delicate young girl. It is something like the reverse of the trick used by professional baseball players who swing two bats while awaiting their turn at the plate.

Consequently, I was unremitting in practicing with my new instruments, using apples, oranges, raw shrimp, my own thumbnail as objects on which to develop an instinctive feel of the mobilizer in my hand. To broaden my hand's experience, I also practiced on dead cats and dogs, and constantly on cadaver heads.

I was a man obsessed. I took specimens to the country so that in the quiet of spring weekends I could work undisturbed. Undisturbed! Early one morning in Katonah, three cars drove up to our door and a small army of New York State troopers and detectives jumped out. With them was a lieutenant of the State Police who identified himself to Helen when she opened the door.

"Where's Dr. Rosen?" he demanded.

"He's sleeping," Helen said, coolly. "What's this all about?"

"You'd better wake him up, Mrs. Rosen," the lieutenant said. "Want to talk to him right away."

Helen doesn't take kindly to being ordered around, least of all by a man whom she regarded as practically personally responsible for the havoc that had occurred at Peekskill a few years before. She looked him over calmly in the way of beautiful women who cannot be intimidated by mere authority.

"Not until you tell me what this is all about, and then *I'll* decide."

"We have reason to believe a homicide has been committed and that Dr. Rosen can give us some information about it," the lieutenant said.

"A homicide!" Helen said, still standing in the doorway so that the officer had to remain outside. "What on earth would Sam know about a homicide?"

"Well, it appears that part of the decedent's body was found on your premises, Mrs. Rosen."

"Part of the body!" Suddenly the light dawned in Helen's mind. "What part? A head?"

"Well, yes, as a matter of fact," the astonished trooper said. "Do you know something about it, Mrs. Rosen?"

"Probably," Helen laughed. "You'd better come in and I'll wake Dr. Rosen. He'll want to handle this himself. Come in the kitchen and have some coffee while I wake him and get dressed."

When I came out, sleepy-eyed and unshaven, there were Helen, a detective, and the lieutenant chatting amiably at the kitchen table while two troopers sulkily drank the proffered coffee at the other end of the table.

Somehow one of my cadaver heads had been taken from the root cellar where I had stored them in crocks. Probably a dog had gotten in and had left it in the tall grass below our lawn. A day or two later, the man I had hired to mow the area with his tractor discovered the grisly object. Naturally, he went straight to the police, who called the District Attorney to inform him that the Red Rosens had been caught at last!

That morning it was not very funny. How was I going to explain it satisfactorily to our visitor without breaking my solemn promise to Mr. "Diener" of Manhattan Medical School?

"I'm conducting a series of experiments with cadaver heads to perfect a new operation that I hope will cure deafness in a very large number of people, perhaps millions," I explained. He listened carefully while I described the operation and the reason why it was necessary to practice it on cadavers. He produced a photograph of the head.

"Recognize it, doctor?" he asked.

"Yes," I said. "That's one of them. Would you like to see the others I have?"

"Where did you get it?" he demanded.

"From the diener of one of the medical schools in New York," I said.

"What's the man's name?"

"I'm sorry, lieutenant," I replied, "but I can't tell you that. I appreciate why you are asking, and I am quite willing to show you other heads that I am using. They are in the garage. But I can't disclose this man's name or the school, because I gave him my word as a physician that I would not give anyone that information, and I won't. It would be highly unethical for me to disclose that."

He looked at me steadily for a moment, then asked to use the phone to call his boss. They talked for a few minutes, and after thanking Helen for the coffee, the men drove off.

Altogether, before I did my first intentional stapes mobilization, I operated on some three hundred cadavers. Sometimes I would make inadvertent mistakes; at other times I would deliberately exert too much pressure, fracturing the crura (the "arms") of the stapes, in order to get the feel of the maximum force that could be safely exerted. At other times I punctured the eardrum by mistake, or dislocated the ossicles, or took down too much or too little of the bony wall of the canal. Each time I erred, I would go to the other ear, or to another cadaver, and *repeat the mistake*, so that I could know exactly how that particular error had been made. Only in that way could I be sure that I would not again inadvertently make the same blunder.

Even these experiments were not enough for my purpose, however, especially in view of the urgency I felt about perfecting this operation, trying it on selected patients, and announcing it to the medical world. I was so intent on what I was doing that I also arranged to perform secret, illegal operations on patients who had just died at several New York hospitals. I bribed the dieners. Why not? I don't regret it for an instant, although there were some ticklish moments when I nearly got caught. Imagine the consequences for a man of my insidiously subversive tendencies. Many a night I was called away from dinner or the theater to attend to "a sick patient"! Since most of those with whom Helen and I socialized had no notion of what an otologist does, they were properly sympathetic to her when the doctor was called away on such "emergencies." Once I left a meeting that was held annually to raise funds to aid the refugees from Fascist Spain. There were pickets outside, carrying signs that declared that people who would help the enemies of Franco were enemies of democracy. It was difficult logic to follow, but there it was. And there they were, when I emerged from the meeting hall. One of the picketers rushed toward me, flailing his sign. He spat in my face and screamed, "You goddam Commie! Why don't you go back to Russia?" I kept on walking, and a policeman stepped between us, waving the angry young ruffian back into the line of pickets. I wiped my face with my handkerchief. If those pickets had had any glimmering of what I was on my way to do, I felt sure they would have tried to kill me. I am convinced that the idea of working with cadavers would have been a sacrilege to them. I felt frightened, assaulted, and angry. As I continued to walk to the corner to hail a cab, a familiar calm settled over me. It was a state of mind I have learned to adopt when some emergency arises in the operating room. I become absolute master of myself, and my mind focuses down on the crisis. At such a moment I can think of a hundred different things—all bearing on the emergency—in a fraction of a second. I can decide what to do and what not to do and in what order to do this and that; and my body, and especially my hands, come under complete control, become the most willing servants of the mind. This time that feeling was centered on the determination that, no matter what the obstacles were, no matter who tried to stop me or interfere with me, I was going to master this operation, devise variations on it, provide for every kind of contingency. There was only so much I could do for those poor souls who had to live in exile from their native Spain because they had fought to support its legally elected democratic government, but here was something I could do in their name, I thought, and in the name of every man and woman who believes in the dignity of man.

Well, perhaps I have gotten carried away a bit here, but it is worth noting that adversity can, as Shakespeare has some character point out, have its good points. This nasty little incident served to strengthen my will to perfect stapes mobilization, just to show them, by God!

There were some close calls in hospital basements. Once I was doing a cadaver operation in the morgue of a certain institution, intent on solving some particular problem. The phone rang, but it distracted me only for an instant. Then it rang again, more insistently. Who the devil would be calling the diener at five in the morning? Suddenly it occurred to me that perhaps it was my friend, the diener, trying to reach *me*. It was.

"Quick!" he hissed into the phone. "Try to put that shroud back the way it was and get out of there fast—and doctor, don't forget to hide your instruments!"

I moved fast—fast enough so that an undertaker and a rabbi who had come for the body never were the wiser. These furtive rendezvous with the recently deceased caused no regret, let alone remorse. Far from doing harm, my work led directly to benefiting millions of men and women, and I cannot for a moment believe that the God of the Jews, Mohammedans, and Christians, if He exists, would disapprove. My cadaver work was done entirely inside the ear. It was quite invisible to any bereaved person looking at the deceased. If it had involved disfiguring the cadaver in any way, I should certainly not have done it. Even after I began to operate on patients, I continued to work on cadavers, because I needed them to maintain my skill, to repeat deliberately mistakes I made in the surgery (of course I made mistakes!), and to experiment with new ideas for overcoming the difficulties that I encountered. I know that my patients derived great good from those witching-hour cadaver operations, and if I am mistaken in my belief that there is no Jehovah, Allah, or God, I am quite prepared to defend myself before Him. But if He exists, I don't think I will have to make any defense. From what I have been privileged to learn of the workings of nature and the universe, it is clear to me that if a deity is involved in it, He is a consummate experimenter Himself.

# Of the Debt
# of the Living to the Dead

Certainly it was not the all-seeing eye of God that watched my midnight adventures and revealed them to the medical director of one hospital where I had made my arrangements with the morgue attendant. Nor was it the Almighty's still, small voice murmuring in the director's ear to the effect that Rosen was up to something down there in the morgue at all hours of the night.

Whatever the motive, I was promptly hailed into the director's presence—and on exceedingly short notice. I was tired and red-eyed from the previous night's subversive explorations of the middle ear of a recently deceased patient in another hospital, or else I would have found myself in serious difficulties. As it was, the director could only indulge in bland insinuations which went approximately thus:

"Sam," he said, batting his owllike eyes at my sleep-filled ones, "people keep telling me that you are awfully busy down at the morgue at all hours of the night. . . . There's a story going around that you are performing some kind of illicit autopsy or some other procedure on recently expired patients . . . "

He let the sentence hang there in the silence of his elegant office. I could think of nothing to say and wisely refrained from uttering some inanity just to fill the silence. As far as I was concerned, I had done nothing wrong, but in spite of myself I felt like a schoolboy who had been summoned to the principal's office.

"It's ridiculous, of course," the director went on smoothly. He was a decent enough fellow, and perhaps he was even more anxious than I not to bring anything out in the open, since such a scandal would probably have caused him more trouble than it would me. "Still, *somebody* has been down there from time to time, Sam, and we can't allow it. None of the funeral directors has complained and there's been no trouble from next of kin, but nevertheless it's completely illegal. Even if a man were to—well, let's say he does some work in the middle ear, something that absolutely doesn't show superficially—even so, we could be held responsible and so could the man who did it. Now, for both his sake and ours I wouldn't want such a thing to happen, so I've given strict orders to the morgue attendants that nobody, but *nobody*, can touch any cadaver brought down to the morgue, except the funeral directors and, of course, the people in pathology performing a duly authorized autopsy."

I still didn't know what to say, so I did the best that an overtired, unimaginative otologist could. "Yes, of course," I said. "I can see that you have no choice, and in your place I would do the same thing, I guess." As I mouthed these platitudes, I began to feel vastly relieved.

"I just thought you ought to know about these absurd rumors," the director went on coolly. "It would be a good idea for all of us to avoid even the *appearance* of doing something that would, uh, lend currency to them."

What a relief! He wasn't going to take any further action.

"Oh, absolutely," I agreed. "What a ridiculous rumor! What on earth will they dream up next?"

"Who knows?" the medical director said dryly. Ostentatiously he began to look through the pile of papers on his desk. It was my exit cue, and I took it with alacrity.

I had a mastoidectomy to do that morning, and as I headed for the operating suite, I thought about the incident. It was politics, I decided. It was just a very serious nuisance, this intramural cold war, nothing more.

It had its effect on me, however. All the attention I seemed to be attracting was giving me a somewhat exaggerated idea of my importance. I knew how dangerous this state of mind can be, particularly for a surgeon. Operating room doors are large and swing open easily to admit both wise men and fools, but I was at least wise enough to know how little I knew and how far I had to go.

The attacks on me had already cut my practice sharply, but that reduction had its compensating feature: when you know there will be precious few patients in your waiting room in the morning, you burn the midnight oil quite freely.

Now I had to find a new source of fresh cadavers. If one hospital director had learned of my activities, others would soon know. I would be shut out of every hospital morgue in the city and the medical school diener was too rich for my depleted financial blood. I had not lost all faith in my colleagues, however, and one of them came to my rescue. He was George Baehr, a Mount Sinai physician and one of the country's foremost experts in community and social medicine. Thanks to this interest, George knew the city health authorities very well indeed. He soon got permission for me to tap a superb source of fresh cadavers: the city morgue at Bellevue Hospital. The willingness of the city health authorities to allow me to do this work saved the day—and not incidentally advanced the development of stapes surgery by months, if not years.

I brought all of my instruments down to First Avenue and 29th Street. The morgue was a fascinating place. It had facilities for hundreds of cadavers. I used to go down every day, sometimes early in the morning, sometimes late at night. At last I had the opportunity to study the middle ear and its structures undisturbed by the possibility of being caught like a naughty boy stealing apples. And study I did. I practiced a variety of techniques. I tried every kind of mistake I could imagine making. I took particular pains to choose cadavers of all sizes, both sexes, all races, so that I would encounter as much variation in middle-ear anatomy as I might expect in the living.

It sounds as if it was a great experience in which the case-hardened surgeon thoroughly enjoyed working on those cadavers, but that is not quite so. Of course it was a tremendous relief to be able to work openly, undistracted by the fear of being apprehended, of being reprimanded, even, perhaps, of having my license to practice suspended by the authorities.

In another sense, it was difficult. Once I got to work with my headlamp, magnifying loupe, and instruments, I could forget about these poor victims of society whose unwanted bodies were mine to practice upon. But late at night in those silent corridors, my thoughts turned upon gloomier matters, thoughts which today no longer disturb me. Perhaps it is the tranquillity which advancing years brings. Nature is sometimes harsh, sometimes kind. Death no longer separates a man from me so sharply as it once did.

When I first entered medical school, I dreaded the gross anatomy lab, where Tony, the diener, presided over the cadavers. I could hardly bring myself to look at the body assigned to me and a fellow student. It was a woman's body and the first thing I noticed about her were the striations across her abdomen, tell-tale whitish lines in the region of the navel. I knew enough medicine even then to realize that they meant that she had given birth to at least three or four children, yet there she was in a medical school morgue, an object for the instruction of two young, irreverent, would-be physicians. All I could think of was, "Oh God, what kind of a world is it, where a woman who has been loved and has given life can die alone, unwanted; and the body that once was a thing of beauty becomes as a cast-off shred of clothing?"

Like many doctors, I had a dread of death and dying. Studies by social scientists have shown that many of us possess an exaggerated fear of death and that we often choose medicine as a way of setting up a psychological defense against this fear. To be a doctor becomes a way of defending oneself and one's fellow man against that terrible enemy. Of course, the practicing physician soon discovers that his knowledge, his skill, and his drugs are a poor shield against that enemy when his patient's time—or his own—has come. He feels utterly powerless, as indeed he is. It is then that he may become something of a menace to the patient and to the family.

In one study at a large California hospital, researchers began with the intention of learning all they could about the attitude of patients toward the fact that they were mortally ill. The researchers were bitterly opposed by the physicians, who were appalled at the idea that their patients might learn that they had terminal illnesses. So the researchers quietly shifted their attention to studying the attitudes of the doctors. The results showed that the physicians were far more disturbed at the prospect of impending decease than the patients. The doctors wanted to make the whole subject absolutely taboo, whereas the patients wished more than anything else that their doctors and nurses would stop pretending that everything was just wonderful and would instead help them deal with the reality that everybody knew was facing them.

Another group of researchers conducted a similar study at my own hospital, Mount Sinai in New York. They confined their scrutiny to patients who were being given intensive radiotherapy for inoperable cancer. As you might expect, the physicians and the radiologists vehemently opposed allowing the research team to discuss the subject of terminal disease with their patients. Not a word was to be said about the nature of the treatment they were receiving or what it signified. In spite of these objections, the psychologists managed to interview patients. They soon discovered that most of them knew perfectly well what the radiotherapy was for and why it would most likely have limited benefits. The carefully kept secret was no secret at all. It was only a comforting illusion being maintained by the doctors, who, of course, sincerely believed that the taboo they had imposed was for the good of their patients.

No doubt many physicians will vigorously deny that they were ever motivated to take up medicine out of such fears. Perhaps so, but I know that it was true in my case. My boyhood fantasies of becoming a doctor were in considerable measure a way of warding off my terror of my mother's asthma attacks. I would discover the cure for asthma and relieve my mother of this frightening malady. My mother would not die, ever, because I would be the all-powerful doctor who would save her.

After a while this daydream was supplanted by a waking nightmare that was the unwanted replay of an accident I had witnessed on a street in Syracuse. I was playing in the street with some other boys. One of them dashed in front of a passing trolley. He slipped and fell under the wheels. The steel rolled over his leg, severing it. Bright red arterial blood spurted from the femoral artery onto the cobblestones. Eventually, an ambulance came and took away his bloodless body, but the gush of blood that had poured from him remained on the pavement and the cold, gray rail where he had lain. The scene was etched in my mind. I could not forget it.

Somewhere along the line I overcame my fear of death and my dread of having to work with the recently dead. Those corpses at Bellevue, many of them dead only a short time, became my friends, my partners in medical research; the winding sheets in which they were wrapped, the uniform of scientific honor. In the autopsy rooms of the world, the dead make a gift to the living that only they can make.

Thanks to our peculiar attitudes toward death, it has long been almost impossible for a living man to decide in advance to make the gift of his body or his vital organs to medical science. For years in most, if not all the states of the Union, only one's next of kin could consent to the disposition of one's body or organs. Gradually this situation is changing, thanks to the passage of a Uniform Anatomical Gift Act by most of the states. The legislation provides that one may, if he chooses, carry on his person a donor card which specifies that his body, or vital organs like the heart or the kidneys, or both (as the person elects) may be used for scientific or therapeutic purposes. Clearly the time is coming when it will be possible with considerable certainty of a good result to transplant the organs of a recently deceased accident victim, for example, to a patient whose life depends upon such a donor. Already cadaver kidneys are being successfully transplanted to living patients. In my judgment, there is no nobler gift that one can make to his fellow human being.

By the same token, the gift of one's body to the next generation of medical men is almost as splendid a contribution to the welfare of those we love, assuming that we do love mankind. Even today, there is a serious shortage of cadavers for study. To some, the thought of making such a gift may be unacceptable, for religious or aesthetic reasons. To others, it may impose too great an emotional burden on surviving relatives. But I like to think that for increasing numbers of Americans this final act of generosity is as natural as the gift of life that springs from the act of love.

# Of the Uses of Skepticism

The living also contribute to medical knowledge and progress. In a law school, students practice their future profession by trying cases in a moot court. In medicine, however, there can be no "moot clinics." Only the living patient can teach the student the complex art and science of healing.

This learning process never ends for competent doctors. Medical knowledge constantly expands. New truths have to be learned, and new errors have to be corrected by demonstrating that they are mistaken estimates of reality. Patients provide the means of doing both. For this reason, no patient, in my opinion, should fail to cooperate when he is being used to teach medical students or doctors. What one of them may learn from observing you may later spare someone else much suffering or even his life. Furthermore, the discussion and consultation that goes on when a patient is used as a teaching case may benefit simultaneously the patient himself and medicine. Two heads are better than one. It happens all the time that an alert house physician or other doctor will note something that the attending doctor has overlooked or failed to realize the significance of.

In medicine, you must never become too old to learn. I was fifty-five years old when Mr. Lawrence came into my life, but in that electrifying moment he opened a new perspective in ear surgery. I did not yet know where it would lead, but I was determined to follow up every possibility.

By the time I had completed my preliminary series of cadaver operations at Bellevue, more than a month had passed since I had mobilized his stapes. Faithfully each week he phoned me from Wisconsin. Each report was good news: he could detect no diminution in the quality and sensitivity of his hearing in the operated ear. He was growing impatient. When, he wanted to know, could he return to New York and let me "do the other one." He was not much concerned about the possibility—still very real—that his sudden access of hearing might be only temporary. As for the risk that the mobilization might ultimately result in damage to the nerve of hearing in the operated ear, he pooh-poohed that completely.

"The ear's absolutely fine," he insisted. "Let's get on with it, please, Dr. Rosen. I'll gladly take my chances on whatever risks there are."

Of course it was gratifying to know how much confidence this intelligent young professional had in my mobilizer and the hand that wielded it, but both scientific and ethical considerations absolutely dictated that I dampen his enthusiasm.

"Now let's take our time on this, Mr. Lawrence," I said. I succeeded in sounding calm, although I was secretly thrilled by the fact that I could speak to him in a normal voice over the wire and know that this patient, who just a month before had to be shouted at, understood me clearly without difficulty.

Mr. Lawrence laughed. "Take our time, take our ti-ycm," he mimicked. For a moment I almost wished his hearing were

not quite so acute! He paused for a moment, and then added
soberly: "Well, I guess I have to go along with you, doctor.
After all, I owe you so much that I guess I owe you a little
patience too."

Patience and patients. The people doctors treat are aptly
named. It was not difficult to understand why he wanted to
"get on with it," and goodness knows, I had no desire to delay
a moment longer than necessary. The longer Mr. Lawrence's
ear remained "new," the greater the likelihood that stapes
mobilization was the answer to many, perhaps most, cases
of otosclerotic deafness. What a boon to millions of the hard
of hearing that would be! But much as I wanted to press ahead
with this exciting new technique, I had a responsibility as a
scientist and as a physician—as a scientist to my profession and
as a physician to my patients. I had to make as sure as I possibly could that no avoidable fault of mine would cause injury
to a patient or falsely raise the hopes of my colleagues that
there had been found a better way to treat conductive deafness
than the ingenious treatment devised by Lempert.

These same two considerations—both demanding delay for
yet a while—had their obverse sides as well. Take the case
for the patient first. Surgical skill is something like athletic
skill. It is acquired only through long, highly disciplined
practice. I knew that I had to develop an exquisitely precise
sense in my hand, something that was more than just muscular
control, something that would be a combination of muscle
sense, touch, feel—call it a pressure sense. It is a difficult thing
to describe, and as difficult a thing to achieve. To develop it,
I resorted to all sorts of devices. For instance, I would peel an
apple fairly thin and place the peel on the ball of my thumb.
Then I would take my needle-sharp instrument and manipulate it with just enough pressure to penetrate the peel. If
I pricked my thumb, I knew I had applied too much pressure,
but if I did not penetrate the peel, it meant that I had not

exerted enough. And all the while I would concentrate as closely as possible on getting the feel of what my fingers, my hand, my wrist, the muscles of my arms were telling my brain as I performed this exercise using apple and orange peels, the carapace of raw shrimp, a crust of bread, a bit of soda cracker.

It was crucial that my brain know precisely what my hand was doing so that I could control its least movement under widely varying conditions. In this way I trained myself not only to control the instrument that would soon be probing the middle ear of a living person but to be totally aware of the resistance encountered by the instrument in relation to the pressure exerted. In other words, by continual practice I taught myself how to interpret all those impulses that were being transmitted along the nerve fibers of my hand and arm to my brain, so that finally I would be able to tell with almost absolute certainty precisely how hard I could press against certain structures with an instrument that weighed a certain amount, that had a certain length, and that had a point of given sharpness or bluntness.

One cannot learn this from reading books or listening to an instructor or even from watching someone else perform the operation. It is learned in the very tissuebed of the fingers, the hand, the forearm. To be certain that I was acquiring this sense of feel for the instrument, I used to practice with my eyes closed —often with apologies to Helen's and my guests—and always I practiced at bedtime for about half an hour in the dark.

No doubt from my description this constant practice sounds tedious but it was nothing of the kind. It was absolutely crucial. The thought of a misstep, of applying pressure needlessly, carelessly, or cumbersomely, and thereby penetrating the footplate of the stapes, haunted me. I had to have absolute control, or I might accidentally invade the dark chamber of the inner ear and do irreparable harm to its delicate structures. And besides, to me the interminable manipulation of the instruments was truly satisfying. I am a surgeon. I was learning to know very exactly how to handle an instrument that no man had ever before handled, and I was getting to know my surgeon's hand as I had never known it before, despite years of experience in the operating room. My nervous system was beginning to integrate the experience as I practiced it over and over. Those muscles and the nervous pathways that controlled them were becoming so interconnected that after a time I could do whatever I wanted within very narrow limits. I could do it blindfolded. In fact, I discovered that by deliberately excluding all other sensations, all other nervous inputs, I could exert even more delicate control and could feel the exact pressure and movements I was making even more precisely.

Now, of course I don't operate blindfolded. The point is that if one can learn to tune his senses to their utmost, a whole world of sensory experience suddenly floods into one's being. For instance, one day I decided to try the same process using taste instead of touch. I was having breakfast. I shut my eyes. I had had bacon, eggs, and toast for breakfast for years, but until that moment I do not believe I ever really tasted them. With my eyes closed I heard the crunching and crackling of the toast in my mouth, felt the mixture of the saliva with the toast until the crunching sounds faded away and the taste of the egg began to predominate along with the lovely sort of burned taste of the bacon. This may sound absurd to the serious-minded. That's too bad—for them. I don't care. There is nothing more delightful than to experience something afresh, like a child. Artists are honored for their capacity to make us see afresh, but we have to be able to look with wonder in our eyes. Great chefs can prepare gourmet foods, but only the diner can, if he will, taste them in all their exquisite variety. Musicians play, but only the trained listener can appreciate the quality and subtlety of the mixture of sounds presented to his ear.

From years of practice, I have concluded that the development of sensory awareness depends upon the ability to experience the sensation in *undiluted* form. One learns to exclude all extraneous mental processes; one never talks in such moments; one thinks only about the sensation or combination of sensations that are relevant. Real art lovers, you may have noticed, stare and stare silently at a single painting on the gallery or museum wall. Watch a concert-goer at a symphony. He is oblivious to his surroundings. Often his lips will be slightly parted because in that way he heightens, ever so slightly, his auditory acuity. His whole attention is concentrated on the sound.

To the surgeon, especially the surgeon who must operate on delicate tissues in confined spaces, the development of this total response to the input of his sense of touch, of his kinesthetic or muscle sense, of his sense of pressures and movement is absolutely crucial.

Another fortnight or so passed. Mr. Lawrence continued to report in by telephone. His hearing remained normal. Morning and night visits to the city morgue reinforced my skills. I had learned to navigate the "perilous ocean" with assurance and deftness. I felt at last justified in going ahead.

Before doing so, however, there was one more river to cross. The series of operations I planned to perform were not just ordinary ones whose reliability, effectiveness, and safety had already been established. They were, despite all of my careful preparation, experimental. Some would perhaps succeed, some would certainly fail. Some would succeed at first, only to fail later. Perhaps even some would be apparent failures at first, only to yield favorable results after a postoperative healing period. It was as if I had explored the land ahead by air, mapped out the route, and prepared everything for the journey, but still had to cross the country on foot, facing unanticipated dangers.

Every competently performed experiment is like such a journey, and every properly written scientific report of such an experiment or series of experiments reveals to its skeptical readers certain essentials: The scientist tells his colleagues the goal of the journey. He describes his preparations for the trip. He provides a detailed map of the route. Then when he embarks, he keeps a detailed log of the expedition into *terra incognita*, describing every step of the way, every difficulty encountered, every "blind canyon" up which he traveled, only to have to turn back and find the main pass through the mountains. Negative results are, to the scientist, as important and as valuable as positive ones, but in our success-oriented society many a researcher finds it particularly difficult to report them. He wants to be able to announce to the world that his goal was California and that he got there from Kansas without once making a misstep. But reality is not like that. Nature gives up her secrets, be they trivial or epoch-making, only very reluctantly. Consequently, competent scientists are, by definition, "strictly from Missouri." They must be shown—especially in medical science, where proof is particularly hard to adduce in a rigorous way. One's fellow specialists are especially insistent upon a thorough, detailed, complete report of every aspect of a new technique, because they are best able to judge what the effect of each step in the process may have been on the results, positive or negative. Besides, once they become convinced of the merit of the procedure, they want to try to replicate it themselves. The only way to convince them that what you have done is effective, safe, and better than the old way is to present the results to them in a large enough number of cases to warrant the belief that the results reported are not the product of mere chance. One swallow, in other words, definitely does not herald the arrival of summer in medical research.

This skeptical, utterly sharp-eyed attitude among researchers, this unwillingness to accept innovation without documentation is the best safeguard against either honest error or outright fraud. It puts up a formidable barrier that protects patients against the widespread use of inadequately tested innovations. So many new ideas eventually prove to be the fruit of hope rather than of fact. Every M.D. hopes to be the one to find something new, ingenious, and useful that will become a part of professional knowledge. We all yearn to have our names attached to some diagnostic sign, some surgical instrument, technique, or operation.

But truth is elusive. Many a researcher has been led down the garden path of his own illusions, imagining that he was on the way to an epochal discovery, only to find that the thorn bush at the end of the path grows no scientific roses. The best protection any investigator or innovator can get against this kind of self-delusion is from his collaborators. Dr. Irvine Page, director of research at the Cleveland Clinic Foundation, is editor of *Modern Medicine* and one of the profession's more pungent commentators. He has remarked that the researcher's best friend is his nearest critic. Far better to expose your cleverest experiments to the skeptical eyes of those who are working with you than to keep them locked up in the laboratory, the morgue, or the operating room, hidden from any objective scrutiny.

I knew this as well as most men, but I was forced to go my own way by most of my associates. They were, if not openly hostile, distinctly cool. I therefore prudently refrained from talking to them about what I was doing. They could hardly be expected to look objectively at my work, I felt. Some, I suspected, might even be capable of trying to appropriate it as their own.

When the long hours in the deadhouse were at last safely past, the time came to work out a strategy that would take into account all these possibilities. The time had come to try to mobilize the stapes of living patients, for which the procedural ground had to be laid with scientific precision. Even the most kindly disposed otologist would rightly insist on incontrovertible proof that stapes mobilization worked, that its effects were lasting, and that the risk to the patient's hearing was minimal —that is, if it worked, and if it proved to be lasting, and if no damage was caused to other organs or structures such as the nerve of hearing or the facial nerve.

One of the most crucial elements of proof had to be a very exact, *totally impartial* testing of the hearing of patients—both before and after stapes mobilization. In the past, I had done this myself, because I wanted to be as sure as possible that each patient was really a good prospect for fenestration. As I have said, fenestration takes a long time to perform, is therefore costly, and results in an ear that must thereafter be treated regularly by an otologist to prevent accumulation of foreign bodies, organisms, and dead tissue at the site of the fenestra. No one would want to subject a patient to all that without first making as certain as possible that he could benefit from it.

The new situation called for a different approach. An audiologist who was completely independent of me and of my hospital was needed to test patients before mobilization and to follow them afterwards. This was essential, not only as a way of providing convincing proof of the merit of the procedure, but also, frankly, as a precaution against possible hostility and bias. If the operations I planned turned out to be only partially successful, I wanted this reported exactly, without distortion. On the other hand, if the results should prove to be very favorable, I wanted to be sure that they were calmly and dispassionately reported in a proper scientific forum.

This problem was not difficult to solve. The name of Dr. Moe Bergman, chief audiologist at Hunter College in New York City, and an audiologist for the Veterans Administration, occurred to me at once. Dr. Bergman's reputation was unassailable. No one could possibly accuse him of reporting results in any but a completely objective fashion. Would he undertake to test patients for me? He would—and without asking what I was up to, either. This had added value, scientifically speaking, for if Dr. Bergman remained innocent, for the time being, of what I was doing, his reports would be, almost by definition, wholly unbiased: he would not know whether to look for improvement in bone conduction or in air conduction; in the high frequencies, the low frequencies, or all the way across the audible spectrum of sound. He would simply compare the patients' hearing at two different times and give me a report of each.

By this time I had performed about three hundred cadaver operations, ironing out all the technical difficulties, learning all the pitfalls of the technique, and perfecting the instruments needed to do the job in any of a score of anatomical variations that I expected to encounter in living patients. I was as ready as I ever would be. The time had come.

# Of Kisses and Gratitude

--------------------------------------------------------------------------

I already knew who would be the first person on whom I would intentionally perform a stapes mobilization. She had been to see me some weeks before, and I had arranged for her return for precise audiometric testing and a thorough examination. Now, with all these preliminaries complete, she sat in my office, looking at me with that slightly apprehensive smile that patients often have at the moment when they know the doctor is going to tell them what he has found.

What I had found was that Mrs. Gray (as we will call her) almost certainly was suffering from otosclerosis. She was sixty and a grandmother. For more than two decades, her hearing had gradually declined, so that she had to use a hearing aid now. She didn't like it.

"I don't mean it isn't better than nothing," she said, "but it just isn't right. I hear so much noise, I guess you'd call it. The hearing aid brings in so much that I don't want to hear, and I think it leaves out a lot that I do want to hear. It's been so long, I can't be sure any more, but isn't normal hearing without an aid very different from hearing with one?"

"Of course," I said. "The best hearing aid is not as good as unaided hearing, just as no set of false teeth can be as good as natural teeth."

When Mrs. Gray was not wearing her hearing aid, you had to talk very loudly, close to her, in order to be understood. She had lost about 50 per cent of her hearing, yet she hated to wear the aid so much that she left it off more often than not. I don't like to shout, any more than anyone else does, so I asked her to put on the hearing aid. Her face fell. She was thinking that I was going to tell her that I could not help her.

I waited while she took the device from her purse and adjusted it. I wanted to be sure she understood everything I was going to tell her, because it was not going to be a simple description of Lempert's fenestration. It was going to be a complicated, detailed description of Rosen's mobilization and of the risks that might be entailed—as well as the advantages—if she consented to the new operation instead of the old one.

"Mrs. Gray, you have the kind of hearing loss that can almost certainly be improved by the fenestration operation you have heard about," I began. "But just recently I have found a different way to operate, a much simpler way, and a much more natural way to try to restore hearing in a case like yours."

There followed an explanation of stapes fixation and stapes mobilization, of my experience with Mr. Lawrence, and (without mentioning cadavers, of course) of my research to perfect the operation.

"Now, this is a new operation," I said. "I feel that it is quite safe and that it may well restore your hearing. But nothing is absolutely safe. There are always some risks in any operation, and in a new one there may be risks that we don't know about yet. And of course it may *not* work, but at least I can assure you of one thing: if it doesn't work, we will only have lost a little time and trouble, you and I, because we will still be able to perform the fenestration operation that I told you about. On the other hand, we can just go ahead with the fenestration, if that's what you would prefer. It's entirely up to you."

It was especially important to be sure that Mrs. Gray clearly understood that the operation was new, that it was untried, and that not only might the results be disappointing but that if we got a good result it might not last. And, indeed, the very act of mobilizing the stapes might conceivably cause some damage to the nerve of hearing in the inner ear, damage that would be irremediable. I went into all of these questions in detail, being careful to make clear that the fenestration would be a more conservative way to proceed, because results were well known and because its reliability was proven by thousands of successful operations. But it was also known that fenestration restores hearing only partially, I explained, whereas my limited, my *very* limited experience with mobilization suggested that it might fully restore natural hearing.

Mrs. Gray smiled at me. Her blue eyes sparkled as she laughed.

"Dr. Rosen," she said confidently, "I may never hear my grandchildren's natural voices if you don't do this for me. Life is short, and I don't expect to live forever, but I would like to live as fully as possible while I'm still able to. Now, why don't we don't we just get on with this and no more discussion of it?"

"Of course we will," I said.

She was an ideal first patient for an untried procedure: mature, intelligent, self-confident. Her 50 per cent hearing loss was already a serious handicap, so that if mobilization proved to be possible, she would regain a dramatic amount of acuity. Above all, she had that quality that you learn to look for in such a situation: a willingness to weigh the advantages against the risks and to decide unequivocally in favor of accepting the risks in the hope of getting the benefits that might accrue.

This was most important, because the opposite side of that coin is a willingness to accept cheerfully, or at least philosophically, the possibility that the operation can fail. If it didn't work, I felt sure, Mrs. Gray was not going to be the kind of patient who turns on the doctor and lashes out at him for his inability to perform miracles.

We scheduled the operation for the following morning. Meanwhile, there was quite a bit to do. I explained about Dr. Bergman.

"Now, for scientific reasons, Dr. Bergman and I would both prefer that you not mention anything to him about the operation. His job is to test your hearing now and then test it again after you have had this new operation."

In the morning when the orderlies and a nurse rolled her into the operating room at Mount Sinai, Mrs. Gray was still smiling. As she was transferred to the operating table, she said nothing, but looked directly at me with those bright blue eyes. I positioned her head carefully and winked at her. We said nothing. Just that wink was enough for her to know that I would do everything that could be done to give her back what she wanted so much. She understood. She winked back, and it was my turn to grin.

It would probably make a better story if I were to tell how, at this point, I was full of misgivings about the new operation: Would it work? Would Mrs. Gray hear again as she once had? Not so. I had practiced and practiced. I had tried every kind of mistake one could make. Mr. Lawrence was still enjoying the full use of his "new" ear. I was sure it would work, and I proceeded confidently to the task of mobilizing Mrs. Gray's stapes, reassuring her about the pinprick of the Novocain needle, incising away the skin of the external canal, lifting the drum, and curetting a bit of the bony wall of the canal so that I had an unobstructed view of the stapes.

It was a familiar territory by now, so familiar that I was

hardly aware that this was a living patient beneath my hands. The ossicles came into view looking like a perfect anatomical model of the middle ear in the magnification of my loupe (see Figure 4). Sure enough, the footplate of the stapes was calcified along the annular ligament. It was a classic case of otosclerosis.

The mobilizer felt comfortable in my hand as I reached in

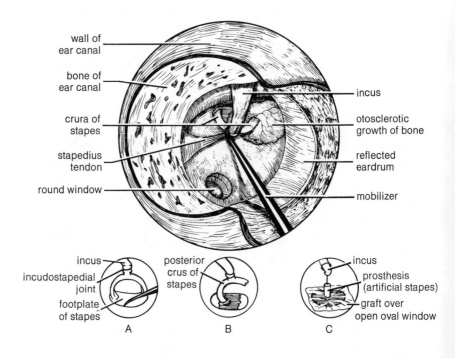

FIGURE 4. *Techniques of stapes surgery. The view through the operating microscope shows the stapes being mobilized indirectly. Diagrams show: A. direct mobilization at the footplate of the stapes; B. radical mobilization, in which a portion of the footplate is removed and the posterior crus serves as a prosthesis provided by nature; C. total removal of the stapes (stapedectomy) and replacement of it by a plastic prosthesis held in place by a tantalum wire attached to the incus. The exposed oval window is covered by a tissue graft.*

and ran its tip up one arm of the stapes until I could feel the depression in the tiny bone that marks the neck of the stapes. This is where it is strongest, as I had proved to my own satisfaction by mounting weights and testing on cadaver stapes.

With the mobilizer I began to pull down on the neck, at first gently, then gradually with stronger and stronger pressure. This was the critical moment. I had to use enough pressure to dislodge the fixated bone in its window, yet not so much force as to fracture the arms. Nothing happened at first. The footplate remained rigidly embedded in the overgrowth of bone. Then, quite suddenly, it began to move, and I eased up on the rhythmic pressure I had been applying to the neck, but continued the pulsating motion of my fingers that would really free the footplate from its diseased moorings. Finally, the lightest pressure resulted in motion. The stapes was free and mobile. Mrs. Gray should hear clearly now.

"Do you hear me, Mrs. Gray?" I whispered.

"Are you shouting?" she asked, her voice muffled by the surgical drapes covering her head.

"No, I am whispering."

She laughed. "If that was a whisper, it sounded like you were talking. It sounds like you've put a loudspeaker down in my ear. For goodness' sake don't talk out loud. Keep whispering, Dr. Rosen, that's plenty loud enough, thank you."

"Well, that's just wonderful!" I exclaimed. "That's great! You've had a successful result."

"For heaven's sake don't talk so loud," she said with evident relish. She couldn't see us, but we were all grinning broadly. If aseptic operating room procedures had allowed it, the scrub nurse and the floating nurse and I would have done a little dance right then and there. Instead, we had to restrain ourselves while I replaced the drum and packed the ear with sterile dressings. Then the nurse removed the drapes and we could permit ourselves the luxury of removing our masks and grinning down at Mrs. Gray while we waited for the orderlies to come with the rolling stretcher.

"Let me kiss you," Mrs. Gray demanded.

Well, why not, I thought, and bent over her. She spontaneously put her arms around me and kissed me. Her eyes brimmed over with tears, but then, there was no dry eye to be seen in that operating room that morning.

Since then I have been kissed in many operating rooms the world over, and not always by gray-haired ladies. Some of them were young and attractive, but that did not stop them from clutching my hand, or throwing their arms around me, or giving me a heartfelt kiss. At Mount Sinai and at the New York Eye and Ear Infirmary, the operating room nurses still tease me about it, but I can defend myself. I don't know a better way than that to get kisses, I always tell them, and they don't argue.

Mrs. Gray's hearing promptly declined just as Mr. Lawrence's had.

"It's as if you had a black eye," I explained to her. "You've probably noticed that it takes a couple of weeks before the blood and the swelling go away and the eye looks normal again. It's the same with your middle ear. It's been pushed and bumped a bit, and it's bled a little, and it will probably take a week or ten days before everything settles down. Now, I am going to discharge you from the hospital in the morning. You go home and relax. Don't let your ear get wet and try not to catch cold and come to see me in ten days at my office."

When I removed the packing ten days later, she immediately noticed the sound of the office air conditioner.

"I never heard an air conditioner before," she said. "You know, Dr. Rosen, even with the packing in I could hear all kinds of new things: jet planes—I never really heard them before, except at the airport—horns tooting, the toilet flushing. And the refrigerator door!"

She laughed: "Maybe my husband isn't going to be so

pleased with you, Dr. Rosen. I found out he sometimes sneaks a midnight snack, even though he's supposed to be on a diet. He got up the other night, and I thought he was going to the bathroom until I heard him open the refrigerator. When he came back to bed, I said: 'George, are you raiding the fridge?'

" 'How did you know?' he said.

" 'I heard the refrigerator door,' I told him, 'and don't slam it so loud next time, either.'

"George is a great tease," Mrs. Gray explained. "He groaned and carried on about nagging wives and we had a good laugh."

I had set up another appointment for her at Moe Bergman's office, and off she went. Within an hour Moe was on the phone.

"Sam!" he exclaimed. "What the hell is going on? I thought you were trying out some new wrinkle on Lempert's or something, but that patient has no sign of any operation at all. Yet she says you operated on her ear. What the hell is going on here, Sam?"

"Wait a minute, Moe," I said. "Back up a little, please. What about the audiogram?"

"You know perfectly well," he said. "Her hearing's normal. No air-bone gap at all. When I tested her, for a minute I thought something had gone wrong with my audiometer, but it calibrates okay. Then I looked up her pre-op audiogram and there was the gap. A fifty per cent loss at least. Come on, Sam! What's it all about?"

Now, Moe Bergman was as disciplined a scientist as any I have ever known, but I could hardly blame him for being excited. The problem was how to avoid telling him without offending him.

"Moe, I haven't gone into it with you because I want to keep this thing as objective as possible. I want your data to be totally uninfluenced by whatever you might think about the work I am doing. That's the right way to do this, it seems to me."

"I suppose so, but—"

"But you would naturally like to know what I am doing, and you will, Moe. I promise. Just go along with me for the first series of patients, won't you please? Then I'll tell you the whole story."

Of course he agreed.

When Mrs. Gray returned a month later, her husband was with her.

"Put the plug back in, doctor," he said. "My lord! The woman hears everything. I, uh, snore a little, it seems, and now she's complaining about it!"

I don't know which of us enjoyed this byplay the most.

"When will you do the other one, Dr. Rosen?" she asked.

"Let's wait and be sure that this one will remain good and won't slip back in any way. I want to be certain of that before we go ahead with your other ear."

The next patient was a practicing attorney. If Mrs. Gray's problem was serious, this man's (we will call him Mr. Brown) was desperate. He was in his late forties and had been having increasing difficulty with his hearing for about fifteen years.

"I'm a trial lawyer, doctor," he told me, "and I love the work. If you can't do something for me, I will have to do something else in law. At times now I can't hear the witnesses clearly. At other times, especially at a conference at the bench, I have a hard time hearing the judge. I think they're saying one thing when they are talking about something else entirely.

"The other day, for instance, the judge called me and the prosecutor up to the bench and began talking about 'incitement.' It made me furious. The idea of his accusing me of inciting anything. It seemed most unfair, and I said so. The judge looked at me in an odd way and said: 'I didn't say anything about "incitement," counselor. I was talking about the third count in the *indictment*.' It turned out that he had decided to instruct the jury to disregard this part of the indictment and wanted to tell me that I need not enter a defense against it.

"You can imagine how embarrassing that kind of thing is, Dr. Rosen. Furthermore, it raises the question whether I can fairly and adequately represent my clients. I practice criminal law almost entirely. I've prosecuted or defended all my professional life, but it looks like I'll have to give it up. I can't conscientiously go on like this. A lot of my clients come into court with a strike or two on them already. They don't need to be handed a cracked bat in the form of a handicapped attorney."

I explained the differences between air-conduction hearing loss and loss due to nerve damage. He understood immediately. Then I examined him and had my audiologist test him. In less than an hour he was back in my consulting room, sitting restively in the chair across from my desk.

"You are fortunate," I told him. "You have the kind of hearing loss that can probably be cured by stapes mobilization."

As I have seen many times before and since, the patient's tension ran out of him like an invisible fluid. He sat back. The lines of his jaw softened. He sighed and looked down at his folded hands. The slight bulging of his eyes and the tautness of the lids vanished, but a tear appeared beneath each closed lid. He blew his nose.

"Damn foolishness, I guess, doctor. But you don't know what a relief it is to know there's some hope."

"That's all it is," I hastened to affirm. "Hope. There are no guarantees in this sort of thing."

"No more than in a courtroom," he said gruffly.

He was as taut as a violin string when he came to surgery a few days later.

"Are you frightened, Mr. Brown?" I asked him, and without waiting for his reply, answered the question. "Naturally, you are. Almost everybody who comes into an operating room is at least a little anxious. Now, of course, in this situation you feel even a bit more tense than usual, because you wonder what's going to be the result.

"Let me tell you something. I am very optimistic about

doing this operation on your ear. Not absolutely certain, of course, but there is every reason to believe that you are an ideal patient for this procedure. So you just relax. You won't be hurt; your chances are very good; and it won't be long now before we'll all know."

He smiled, not very certainly, but he put a good face on it. Who could blame him for being terribly concerned? His whole professional future hung in the balance in that operating room that morning.

Like Mr. Lawrence and Mrs. Gray, the lawyer's hearing came back as I mobilized his stapes.

"Doctor," he said from beneath the drapes. "I can hear everything that's going on. A moment ago you asked your assistant if she had cotton ready. Were you speaking loudly then?"

"No, Mr. Brown. Just in an ordinary tone of voice."

"It sounded as if you were shouting," he said happily.

A few days later, when he came to my office, I knew at once that his hearing loss had been eliminated. With the packing removed he could hear normally in the operated ear. In fact, his hearing was perhaps a little more acute than my own, for he could hear one of my nurses talking to the audiologist in the waiting room.

He too went to Moe Bergman for testing, of course, and again the results were strikingly positive. This time, however, it was my turn to be curious, because Moe did not phone me after performing the audiology on the lawyer.

"Same thing, Sam," Moe said when I phoned him. "No use asking you what you're up to yet, is there?"

"Let's play it this way for a while, Moe," I said.

"It's your baby," he said. "And it's some baby if this keeps up one after another."

"Well, we'll have to wait and see," I said. "Besides, I'm going to ask you to do follow-up testing on all of them."

"Only proper way to go about it," he said. It was good to hear him talk that way. Nothing could be worse for everyone concerned than for the investigators in such an experimental series to let their enthusiasm carry away their judgment.

A month later Mr. Brown was back for another checkup and regaled me with tales of the courtroom—not the legal level but the auditory. The day before, a recalcitrant witness had muttered something in response to a question, and the judge had said sharply: "Speak up, Mr. Witness."

" 'He answered in the negative, Your Honor,' I told him.

" 'Thank you, Mr. Brown,' the judge said. Then he did a double take, and so did I, because we both realized that he was the one with whom I had had the misunderstanding about 'incitement' only a few months ago.

"After court, he asked me what had happened, and of course I told him all about you, doctor. I wish there were some other way I could thank you for all that you've done."

"You just go on using that new ear of yours," I said. "And take a few sensible precautions about it. Don't swim for, say, two or three months—make it three months, do you mind? And try to avoid catching a cold. If you do, don't blow your nose, just wipe it with a tissue, and if it threatens to be a bad cold, pretend, if you will, that you're really sick and go to bed and take no chances. If an infection should get into your middle ear, you see, it might sabotage our results.

"You do those things for me and for yourself and that will be more than enough thanks. Then in six months, come back so that I can test your ear again, will you please?"

"Anything you say, doctor. I'm really so grateful I can't put it into words."

"Well, I'm pretty grateful to you, Mr. Brown, if the truth be known," I said as we shook hands. He looked puzzled, but I didn't enlighten him.

# Of the Abuses of Skepticism

That made two home runs out of two times at bat. After each operation I had to go to my office and see patients. Then I would perhaps go down to Bellevue to practice some more on cadavers before going home. But each time I could hardly wait to tell the good news to Helen, my daughter, Judy, and son, John.

They had shared both the good things in my life and the bad. At dinner on the night of Mrs. Gray's operation, I told them just what had happened. Judy jumped up from the table and flung her arms around me and kissed me. (More kisses!)

"Oh, Dad, it's just super," she exclaimed, and then added a thought that is typical of her: "It's so good to be able to give someone so much happiness."

Helen and John were just as pleased.

"Knowing you," Helen said, "there won't be any getting you to say that this is a success yet, will there?"

"Not outside this house," I said, "but between the four of us let's say it works, at least in three cases."

That was as far as I was willing to go, even in the bosom of my family. It was all very well to be enthusiastic, even exultant, but the road ahead might be full of pitfalls. There was, first of all, the crucial question of how long the improvement would last. To find that out, I had to steel myself to wait patiently while time inched along and my patients, bless them, faithfully returned to Dr. Bergman and to me for retesting of their hearing.

Then there were other unpleasant possibilities. Perhaps mobilization, in time, turned out to be damaging to the inner ear and its delicate nerves. If so, the technique would have to be abandoned. Or perhaps there would be patients whose stapes was so rigidly fixed that the "arms" of the stapes (the crura) would fracture before enough pressure could be applied to render the footplate mobile and restore hearing.

One thing was very reassuring. If the crura of the stapes were fractured during the procedure, all was not lost. The patient, still with an immobile stapes, could be given usable hearing by fenestration. This fact emboldened me when I began to encounter cases in which the cautious pressure of the mobilizer that I had at first applied proved insufficient to loosen the footplate in its bed of calcified overgrowth. It seemed safe to press harder, especially as my skills became surer and my knowledge of anatomical differences broader.

It was not long before I had a dozen cases to my credit. Some were more successful than others. Some patients, for instance, did not have purely conductive hearing loss, but a mixture of conductive and perceptive—i.e., nerve—loss. These patients could benefit from stapes mobilization only to the extent that their loss was due to otosclerosis rather than to the loss caused by deterioration of the nerve of hearing. But often the improvement was enough to make all the difference in the patient's life.

Naturally, I kept meticulous notes of each case so that, as

the time passed, I would be able to re-examine every detail of each operation—exactly what I found in the preoperative testing and examination, precisely what I did during the operation and what happened afterwards, exactly what the postoperative test results were, what the longer-term results were, and so on. Only in this way was it gradually possible to decide what kinds of methods were best suited to different kinds of situations, and, for that matter, what methods I had tried gave poor results.

Of course the otologists at the hospital heard about what I was doing. I was in the operating room performing stapes mobilizations more and more often. At first no more than one every ten days or so, but gradually the number of cases increased. And what was happening to the fenestrations? They disappeared from the operating room schedule—at least they did so opposite my name on the schedule. It just read: "Rosen —ear surgery for otosclerosis." Then the patient's name; then the assigned operating room. It got around, I am sure. Rosen would go into the operating room for what ought to have been a two-hour procedure, but he would be out in half an hour, wearing his street clothes and going on rounds to see his patients. What the devil was the fellow up to, anyway? The gossip began to echo up and down the white-tiled corridors of the operating suite—and along the passageways.

A hospital has a life of its own that is different from that of any other kind of institution. For one thing, the doctors in it are marvelously autonomous. I am used to this myself. Here are literally millions upon millions of dollars' worth of plant and equipment at my disposal, all paid for by the patients, the city, the state, the federal government, and, of course, philanthropists. All this, and a staff of nurse's aides, orderlies, practical and registered nurses, interns, residents at the behest of the attending physician, surgeon, radiologist, etc., who dispose of these marvelous facilities and the salaried staff who man them as we, in our licensed wisdom, shall decide is best for our patients.

The arrangement inevitably gives us a sense of power and a certain self-satisfaction about our unique status. We cannot be ordinary men, if society places at our disposal such costly resources while leaving us free to exact whatever we wish in the way of fees for our services, most of which, especially in the case of surgeons, can only be rendered in the hospital.

Consequently, among the attendings, a special kind of élitism develops. We are a breed apart, and furthermore, given the specialization in medicine and surgery, each branch, twig, and twiglet becomes a kind of private club. The neurologists talk to the neurologists, the gynecologists to the gynecologists, the thoracic surgeons to the thoracic surgeons, the cardiologists to the cardiologists, and, of course, the otologists to the otologists. We nod to each other as we hasten along the corridors; we even speak to each other across the bed, as we consult one another about the diagnosis and treatment of a particular patient prostrate between us and, as we correctly suppose, entirely dependent upon our decisions, for there is very little Patient Power in the modern American hospital.

As I accumulated cases, I became ever more convinced that stapes mobilization was a genuine breakthrough. Not epoch-making, like Harvey's discovery of the circulation of the blood, but, nevertheless, a new technique that potentially could restore millions of persons who were handicapped by hearing disabilities to the full *natural* hearing they had once enjoyed. Underscore that word *natural*. Of course there was no way for me not to start telling my colleagues about what I had discovered. On the contrary, I wanted them to know. They were still doing fenestrations, for heaven's sake, and here was something they should know about and look at. For that matter, they should also tell me what was wrong with it, if anything was, so that I could get the benefit of their cautionary observations of my work while their patients could benefit by having a go at a simpler, more natural way to overcome the disability imposed by otosclerosis.

Remember that I had worked for a quarter of a century by then. We were all on the ear, nose, and throat service of Mount Sinai. At least two or three colleagues had been there with me during all that time.

"I want to tell you what I am up to," I said to one of them. "You and I know how difficult fenestration is. Not very many men can do it. Apparently I have sort of stumbled into something that is a lot simpler."

He listened while I told him of my experience with Mr. Lawrence. By then three or four months had passed, and my engineering friend had dutifully called me each week to say that his new ear was as "new" as ever. It was still turning in reports from the outside world as clear and as authentic as when he was a boy.

"I thought maybe that was just a fluke," I said, "but since then I have done a dozen more. Of course, meanwhile I went to the morgue and studied the whole thing out very carefully on cadavers, you understand. Even had a special set of instruments made for the procedure. I've done maybe three hundred cadaver operations.

"Look! I've already done a dozen operations, but more are coming in all the time. Some of them are patients who are referred for fenestration, only I don't do that any more. I don't need to. This operation takes only a few minutes, causes practically no vertigo or other symptoms of disturbance in the labyrinth, and is so untraumatic that I can discharge the patient the day after the operation.

"Now, why don't you come and see the next series of patients? Test them yourself. See them during the operation. Watch what I do and let me show you, step by step, how I do it, and then follow them afterwards. You can have your own audiologist test them."

He sipped his coffee calmly. One would have thought that we were just idly passing the time in the hospital cafeteria.

Looking at him, an observer would suppose that nothing of any importance whatever was being discussed. He said nothing.

"Tell you what," I said. "Today is Tuesday. On Thursday I have another case. It's on the schedule. If you can come, I would be really tickled to have you, because I want you to see this. Maybe this one won't be successful, but I want you to see what I'm doing."

He never came.

"Sorry, Sam, I was tied up and couldn't make it," he said.

"That's all right," I said. "I know how it is." But of course I did *not* know how it was. How could anybody, I wondered, miss a chance to see a thing like this? Here was a potential revolution in the whole field of surgery for conductive deafness, the very specialty that he was most vitally interested in, but he let an appointment get in the way of being a part of it.

"I'll let you know when the next one is scheduled," I promised.

When the next mobilization was set, I called his office and left word of the time and the operating room.

"I'd appreciate it if the doctor would let me know if he plans to be there," I told his secretary.

He didn't come. He didn't call. I could not really understand this, especially from an old friend, but I shrugged it off, even the palpable discourtesy of his not telling me that he would not be able to be present. Perhaps he thinks the whole thing is illogical, or theoretically impossible, I argued to myself. But I could not really believe that a man with whom I had worked side by side, with whom I had shared many a tough clinical or surgical problem, would not do me at least the elementary professional courtesy of coming to see something new and potentially of major importance to our specialty.

It was a busy time for me. There were not enough patients for the new operation to permit me to abandon cadaver work. I had to keep my hand in, and so I often repaired to the morgue.

I thought of new possibilities, new variations on this exciting surgical theme, and I always tried them out on the dead, not the living. I didn't bother my head much about my erstwhile friend, any more than I spent much time worrying about the same reaction from another old associate who had been on the service with me for two decades or more. I went over the same story with him, but by now I had learned something.

He asked no questions, made no comment, but I went on doggedly.

"I have one scheduled for Monday and another one on Friday," I said insistently. "I want you and the men in our hospital to have a look at this thing. Come and test it, test the patients before and after, look at the procedure, accept it or turn it down, approve it or disapprove it.

"I want you to take over the patients before the operation. Test them, then watch me perform the operation, then test the patients afterward and follow them for a month, six months, a year. No monkey business, you understand? You control the whole thing, so there can be no question of what I do and what the results are."

He just stared at me with a funny, half-derisive smile on his face. It was not a happy moment for him, now that I look back on it. His pupils were dilated as if he were undergoing some kind of internal panic. He gulped.

"Of course, of course," he said. "I'll do my best to be there."

And of course he did not show up, either on Monday or Friday. The next time I ran into him in the surgeons' dressing room, I stood between the lockers so he could not pass. He would have had to push me aside to get by.

"Listen," I said. "I don't know what the hell is bothering you guys on the staff, but I don't give a good goddamn any more. To hell with the whole bunch of you, the chief of the service included."

I was absolutely outraged, and I guess I raised my voice

in a most undoctorly manner. "You don't seem to understand that I have a fact in my hands. Do you know what a fact is? It contradicts whatever stupid opinion you and the chief and the others may have. If I ignored it, it would brush me aside too. Are you going to look at it, or are you going to shut your eyes? Are you afraid it might be true? What the hell is the matter with the lot of you?"

He never said a word. He just stood there in his underwear staring at me with that funny, crooked smile, half ashamed, perhaps, but the other half superciliously laughing at me, as if that were somehow going to change anything at all.

"Oh, the hell with the whole lot of you and the hospital too! Who needs you? I don't."

Still, I couldn't quite believe it. I kept trying to interest them. I called my best friend who was also on the Mount Sinai service. Somehow he couldn't find time either, though I told him well in advance when an operation was scheduled.

"Well, I don't know if I can make that one," he kept saying over and over like a broken record.

"Tell you what," I said. "You tell *me* when you're free, and I'll shift a patient around, or postpone his surgery or something so that you can see what I am doing."

Never a word from him, needless to add, nor from other attendings, some of whom I had trained as residents. Not one would come to see this work.

When I told Helen about all this kerfuffle, she laughed sympathetically. "You've got a case of scarlet fever, Sam," she said.

I knew at once what she meant. A man likes to tell his wife stories about his days as a young man. Helen was referring to my first patient and what had happened.

I was a student at Syracuse Medical School. One of our duties was to make emergency house calls, and the first one that I was sent on was to a shanty where a child lay ill in a darkened room. I asked the mother to bring the feverish child over to the window so that I could at least examine as best one could under those conditions. As soon as she brought the child into the light, I could see that he had a rash, but I had no notion how to interpret it. After I left the house, I racked my brains to unearth some tidbit of medical wisdom that would lead me to a correct diagnosis, but I remained as much in the dark as the child had been. So I did what any right-thinking boy would do: I called my mother and described the child's symptoms to her.

"He's got scarlet fever," she said with total conviction.

Returning to the medical school, I reported the case. It was a serious matter in those days. Scarlet fever was highly contagious and was known to cause serious secondary illnesses, such as rheumatic fever, including damage to the valves of the heart. Doctors, real doctors, were dispatched at once, and in short order the shanty was placarded with quarantine signs: KEEP OUT! SCARLET FEVER! BY ORDER OF THE BOARD OF HEALTH. Every day for the next two or three weeks I used to walk to medical school via a detour that took me past that wonderful quarantine sign that confirmed my diagnosis. It was fantastic. Think of it: scarlet fever! And Sam Rosen had diagnosed it. If I had ever doubted that I was going to be a good doctor, those doubts were dispelled.

Thirty years later, the doctors at Mount Sinai discovered a new disease entity. Apparently "Rosen Fever" was even more contagious than the "scarlet" kind, because not a single member of the staff dared venture past the invisible quarantine placard on my operating room door.

# Of Courtesy,
# Courage, and Cowardice

---

Patient after patient underwent stapes mobilization in the Mount Sinai operating room. Earlier efforts to have me removed from the Mount Sinai staff as a "dangerous Communist" or something had failed. It was still "my" hospital, and I still had the right to admit patients and operate on them there. I also had the right to make my feelings known to the superintendent. I stood just inside the closed doors of his huge office, an enormous paneled room containing a desk the size of a double bed. It was quite a job to get an appointment with him, but I waited patiently enough to be shown in to the presence. Once inside, I didn't waste my time. I described the strange indifference of the entire ear, nose, and throat staff.

"I've always felt it was best to keep things in the family," I said. "I don't mean just family quarrels. I mean the good things, too. Our own people should have the first chance to judge this new development, and, if they think it has merit, to learn how to do it."

He listened coldly and finally said: "Well, Sam, you can't force people to come to see what you're doing. What do you want me to do, anyway?"

Would the possible fame that the hospital might acquire have any influence on him? Probably not, I decided. Mount Sinai's reputation was superb. It needed no special recognition, though I felt sure that my work would enhance its reputation. The trouble was that it would also enhance mine.

"If we just pretend Rosen and his funny ear operation don't exist," they seemed to be saying, "they will both go away and we won't have to worry any more about our status, our patients, and our standing with the board of trustees, and our comfortable certainty that, in performing expensive fenestration procedures, we are really doing the best for our patients."

But that rascal Rosen wouldn't oblige. One of the things he did was to drag the whole embarrassing business into the monthly E.N.T. staff conference. This was a group of about fifteen men from the attending staff and the out-patient department who got together regularly to discuss the operation of the E.N.T. service, present interesting cases, debate the diagnosis of a puzzling case, and in general exchange ideas and muted criticism.

By that time I had done stapes mobilizations on perhaps a score of patients. I arranged for five or six to appear and explained to the conference what I had done to them.

"Gentlemen," I said. "I invite you to examine these patients. Take an otoscope and look in each ear. You won't be able to tell which one was operated on in some cases, because most of them had this surgery months ago. But if you look at the preoperative audiograms and if you care to use these tuning forks, you can determine for yourselves that there has been a marked improvement in hearing. In some cases it is only a partial improvement, in others the hearing in the operated ear is now normal."

Did the doctors assembled spring with alacrity to their feet? No. Did they rush to grab the otoscope, snap on the light, and peer into the ears of my patients? Not one of them. Did they so much as touch those forks to perform a Rinne or a Schwabach test? Not a soul.

There was dead silence. The chief of the service, who always presided at the monthly conference, was stony-faced. The men looked at him, and he stared back absolutely expressionless. Slowly they got to their feet and examined the patients. With almost painful reluctance, they forced themselves to inquire into what was for each of them an unwelcome but nonetheless revolutionary development in the specialty of their choice. They were witnessing a turning point in the history of their specialty. They were at the continental divide of their life's work in their chosen field, yet they approached the patients with all the eagerness of condemned men walking to the executioner's outstretched arms.

It had occurred to me, of course, that my audience might persist in its skepticism. To counter this a bit more, I had come prepared with another exhibit. Two days before the conference, I had gathered up all the tiny incus bones that I had removed from cadaver ears. The incus, you will recall, is the bone that articulates with the stapes. After completing my work with each cadaver I had removed the incudes and preserved them in formalin. By now I had hundreds. I counted them on the table in my bedroom where I keep my microscope. How many would be convincing to these people? I asked myself. Never mind. I was satisfied, and put them in a pill bottle.

"It seemed just possible," I said, "that you might not be quite convinced that I have been doing so much work on this operation. Actually I have done hundreds of cadaver operations in order to perfect it, and I want to show you the proof."

I held up the bottle.

"If anybody would care to count the incudes in this bottle,

he will be able to certify that there are exactly one thousand."

No response.

"Well," I continued, "I'm almost done. Let me tell you something: You're all going to have to face this fact whether you like it or not. It just won't go away, and neither will I. You've had your chance to take this up, look at it, test the patients, learn the procedure. You obviously don't want to. You're obviously afraid of something that's new, but sooner or later you're going to have to come to terms with it. Otherwise you will miss a big, important thing. That's what this is, and you're letting yourselves be left out in the cold because you're afraid."

No response to that little speech either. I gathered up my equipment, thanked my patients, and left. I am not a tall man, but when I walked out of the room, I felt a head taller than any man present. They were so unscientific, so profoundly biased that they tried to ignore the whole thing rather than see it grow and develop in the hands of someone they had been told was unworthy. Why, they were so paralyzed that they would not even attack me.

I never consulted these men again, never asked them to witness a mobilization, never discussed the subject with them. They were a lost cause. I decided to face this unpleasant fact and turn elsewhere for scientific criticism of my work, for no man in research can safely stand alone with a new departure in treatment. He needs the genuine, searching scrutiny of his colleagues to keep him in line, to keep him from becoming infatuated with his own discovery and thus losing sight of its dangers and its limitations.

And of course he needs recognition of his achievement. I decided the time had come to present the results of my preliminary work before the section on otolaryngology for the New York Academy of Medicine, of which I had been a fellow for about a quarter century.

Strangely enough, the program committee of the section could never find time to let me present a paper. One day on Park Avenue I ran into a member of the committee and asked him why it was that there never seemed to be any opening for me. He was very uncomfortable. It was because I didn't attend all the meetings, perhaps (as if anyone ever did!). *He* was very anxious to have me present this new thing, but, uh, others were, well, not so eager. Perhaps the committee could be persuaded to put me on the program at some later date, he suggested, and hastened on his way.

Meanwhile, events were moving swiftly. Although my colleagues solemnly and officially pretended that nothing was happening in my Mount Sinai operating room, behind my back they were gabbling about "Rosen's thing" like a gaggle of geese. I knew that sooner or later some bold soul would try to mobilize a patient's stapes. He might succeed and then try to take the credit for it. Worse, he might fail and perhaps injure his patient irreparably. This would discredit the procedure before it had a proper trial. Determined not to let this happen, I telephoned the chairman of the Section on Ophthalmology and Otolaryngology of the Medical Society of the State of New York, Dr. Benjamin Volk of Albany. I told Dr. Volk the whole story, the Lawrence operation, the hundreds of cadaver experiments, the successful operations that followed.

"We've already published the program for the May meeting of the section in Buffalo, Dr. Rosen," he said, "but this is awfully exciting. I think you ought to present it right away, so tell me: How long a paper do you want to read?"

"I can read it in ten minutes at most," I assured him.

"Fine," Dr. Volk said. "I will just add you to the end of the program and introduce you myself."

It was the 147th annual meeting of the section, and it was one of the most important days in my life. I prepared for it carefully. The doctors would want to know the whole story.

And that was what I gave them, as completely and honestly as I knew how.

The first part of my presentation recalled our successes with fenestration surgery. Fenestration is done, I said, because fixation of the stapes "is assumed to be permanent and irreversible, hence the necessity for creating a new window which permits sound to reach the cochlea more readily." I had my audience right with me on that. We all knew this was absolutely true. It was otologic gospel. But then I went on:

> The purpose of this preliminary report is to present evidence that in otosclerosis the fixed footplate of the stapes in the oval window may be rendered freely movable by manual manipulation with a probe through the external auditory canal. By thus restoring the normal mechanism and function of the intact ossicular chain, improved and even normal hearing has resulted.

If anyone had been bored up to then, they were so no longer. I was flatly declaring that there was now something simpler and sometimes even better than the long, costly, and only partially curative procedure they had all been using. Would they really believe me? I did not know, but they were entitled to a full, frank disclosure of precisely how stapes mobilization was done and of the results. I gave them just that: I described the operation in detail, illustrating it with slides and audiograms. Lest they doubt the strength of the stapes, I showed them my photograph of an 8-ounce pharmacist's weight suspended by a wire from the neck of a cadaver stapes, assuring them that not only was the force exerted by the surgeon applied in a similar direction but that it was considerably less than 8 ounces.

Then came the details of five cases. In two, the patients had recovered normal hearing; in three, hearing had improved, but to less than normal because mobilization had not closed the air-bone gap, or because the patient's hearing by bone conduction was below normal in the first place. In each case, I emphasized, the operation was simple; the patient was able to leave the hospital on the following day; he suffered no ill effects, such as dizziness; and in marked contrast to fenestration surgery, he required no postoperative care. Furthermore, the good results had lasted as long as a year.

When I had finished, silence greeted me. My heart sank: these men in Buffalo were going to be like all the rest. Dr. Volk began to speak. A short, graying man with a kindly face and sharp, bright eyes, he thanked me and turned to the assembled doctors:

"I took the liberty of adding Dr. Rosen to the program," he said, "because it seemed to me that what he had to tell us was of importance to the profession. Now that we have heard him, it seems to me to be so remarkable that we should allow an unlimited period for discussion and questions. The floor is now open for that purpose."

A hand flashed. Well, at least they were going to react, I thought, and braced myself for whatever might come, be it hostility, skepticism, curiosity, or acceptance. I need not have worried. They pounded me with searching questions, the very ones I had already asked myself in the deadhouse, in the operating room, and in anxious consultation over Moe Bergman's audiograms of these and other patients. They were the questions that any serious, scientific mind would raise: Why does this work? How does it work? Why doesn't the stapes break under such pressure? How much pressure will it stand before fracturing? Isn't the procedure dangerous? Might it not injure the cochlea, the inner ear and its delicate nerve mechanisms? And practical questions: How do you see what you are doing? How do you expose the incus and stapes enough to have a field of vision and room for manipulation?

In the group of about fifty men, there were perhaps only

four or five who performed Lempert fenestrations. The rest restricted their practice to other treatment of the ear, nose, and throat. But after the discussion period, a dozen men gathered around me to ask more questions, mostly detailed inquiries about exact fine points of technique. I answered them as fully as possible, but there was one thing that worried me in particular:

"You have to practice this thing thoroughly on the cadaver before you try it," I told them. "It looks deceptively simple, but I urge you to do at least fifty cadaver operations before you try this on a patient. Otherwise the risk of making a mistake is very high."

I was so concerned about this that I invited them to come to New York and watch me work and to do a few cadaver operations at Bellevue with me.

"Is there a fee, Dr. Rosen?" a surgeon who had studied under Lempert asked quietly.

"No," I said. "There is no fee. Pay your own expenses, and that's all it will cost you."

When we were finished, I looked around the room for a man I had spotted in the audience. I am not going to mention his name, because what happened in those years is over and done with. I suppose he came to the Buffalo meeting because it was convenient. In any event, he had sat unmoving in his chair throughout my presentation and the question period that followed. He never batted an eye; never made a comment; never asked a question. Now he was gone. Perhaps he had had no time to stay on, I thought, and so I sent him a copy of the paper, a set of audiograms, and the drawing and photographs I had prepared. Later I sent him a reprint of the paper as it appeared in the *New York State Journal of Medicine,* and as I published one paper after another about stapes mobilization, I continued to send him reprints of my articles. For a long time there was no response, but then there came a letter saying that he did not care to receive any additional reprints from me and asking me to strike him off my list.

I answered promptly. Naturally I would send him no further reprints, I wrote. I told him that I regretted that he had evidently formed an unfavorable opinion of me, but there was nothing I could or would do about that. As a matter of fact, I added, his discourtesy and his refusal to look objectively at the facts about stapes mobilization had forced me to come to rather negative conclusions about his merit as a scientist, although I still regarded him as among the most highly skilled of technicians in ear surgery.

He did not reply. As before, we would encounter each other three or four times a year at meetings in the United States and Canada. He had always looked through me on these occasions, as if I did not exist, but from then on, it was mutual. We were invisible otologists, made of so much plate glass as we passed each other in hotel corridors or meeting room aisles: not a nod or a word, just a stony stare at the wall behind each of us.

# Of Honor Abroad

Now that I was on the record, I could work even more deliberately. It would no longer be possible for someone to perform a series of mobilizations and then claim that he had devised this new technique. But the continued hostility toward me remained. Back in New York City, everyone knew that I had at last delivered my preliminary report. Stapes mobilization was now, for all time, the Rosen mobilization.

The game took a new turn. My colleagues conceded that the Rosen mobilization existed, but it was dangerous. It deafened patients. It caused permanent damage to the nerve of hearing, so that the unfortunate victim of Rosen's irresponsible experimentation emerged worse off than ever. Besides, Rosen, who has been having a justifiably hard time with his practice thanks to his Communist proclivities, charges fantastically exorbitant fees for his simple-minded sleight of hand. Furthermore, there is really nothing to the procedure. Any intern can do it—not that he should, because it is both ineffective and extremely dangerous. And so on and on . . .

But I had other things on my mind. The most important was that, using the technique I had begun with, only about three out of ten patients could be mobilized successfully. The rest had stapes that were so firmly embedded in overgrowth of bone that when I tried to mobilize them either nothing happened at all or the crura fractured, sometimes with an audible crack. This was not too frightening, since it was always possible to bring the patient back later for a fenestration.

It was disappointing, however. I was sure that mobilization was the most natural way to restore hearing in these cases, and I was determined to find ways to restore the natural function. I began to ponder the possibilities for approaching these more stubborn cases, but the answers were slow in coming. At the time, however, I was too busy dealing with an accumulation of cases and with the reaction to my announcement of the stapes mobilization. There were, after all, some colleagues who were interested.

In gradually increasing numbers, they came to Mount Sinai to watch me work and accompanied me to Bellevue, where they performed cadaver operations under my eye. But it was slow, so slow that I decided to test the truth of the adage that "A prophet is not without honor save in his own country." In other words, I decided to travel abroad, teaching stapes surgery and hoping that the foreigners would pay more attention than my fellow Americans. If some Canadians were hostile, would the English be? If my colleagues at Mount Sinai were ice cold, would those in Tel Aviv and Haifa be the same?

As I write this, it is difficult to recapture those first experiences abroad. By now I have taught ear surgery in so many countries that I have literally lost count. The number is at least forty and the cities, the doctors, the hospitals, the operating rooms, the nurses, the patients are all blended in my mind into one vast, colorful array of humanity.

But in 1953 it was different. I arranged to visit Mr. Terence, later Sir Terence, Cawthorne, who was England's most distinguished ear surgeon.

Mr. Cawthorne was a gentleman of great eminence in English medicine. His offices on Harley Street were understated in a characteristically British way. His consulting room was, by comparison with those occupied by most Park Avenue specialists, small and sparsely furnished. The walls were mahogany. There were two ample chairs of black leather at either corner of his desk, behind which he sat in a well-used swivel chair. The other rooms were equally unpretentious. In truth, they were ostentatiously unpretentious and produced just the desired impression of a man who had attained such status in his world that mere amenities no longer concerned him beyond their immediate practicality. This style was one that I happened to like.

Sitting in Mr. Cawthorne's consulting room, however, I was not completely at ease. He was very courteous. For perhaps two hours he listened politely, even attentively, to my description of stapes mobilization, looked at my records, at audiograms, at the details of cases. Occasionally he looked at me with just a hint of speculation in his glance, as if he were thinking: "Who is this fellow? I've read his papers in the journals, but who is he really? Some American medicine man, perhaps? Some purveyor of a new kind of snake oil to delude the unwary into false hopes of an easy cure for conductive deafness?"

He listened and listened and listened. Every once in a while I would pause and an uncomfortable silence filled the room.

Finally, I said bluntly: "Mr. Cawthorne, you don't seem to be terribly impressed by all this."

"Oh, not at all," he answered with grave courtesy. "I'm really most impressed, Dr. Rosen, most impressed."

Somehow, it did not ring true. If he had been so interested

and had found my work so worthwhile, why wasn't he commenting? Why wasn't he asking me all sorts of practical and theoretical questions about it? It seemed to me that he was just tolerating my presence, maybe even thinking about something else entirely, perhaps planning a fenestration operation he would be doing the next day. It infuriated me. Here I was getting the same treatment that I had received at home, except for a few men who had their eyes and minds open enough to see what all this really meant. This Englishman, I thought, is as bad as all the rest of them. He's so married to Lempert's fenestration that he can't even consider seriously what I am trying to tell him. And to top it off, he's so damned gentlemanly and polite and so very, very British. Well, I would unruffle this calm.

"Let me suggest something, Mr. Cawthorne," I said. "Perhaps you have a suitable patient right now, or perhaps we will have to search for one. It doesn't matter. You will keep complete control of the patient. All I ask is that the indications be unequivocally diagnostic of otosclerosis—normal bone conduction, air-bone gap, that sort of thing. You test him as thoroughly as possible before surgery. Then, on the patient of your choice, I will do this operation here in London. Afterward, you can follow the patient's progress and draw your own conclusions."

The instant I launched upon this proposal, I realized that I had been thinking very unkind thoughts about Mr. Cawthorne. He sat up in his swivel chair, put his elbows on his desk, and riveted his attention on me. His eyes came alive. He breathed more rapidly. Here was no timid or self-seeking practitioner who feared the prospect of giving up his time-consuming, lucrative fenestration operations. Behind the Britisher's reserve was a bold, imaginative mind. The thought of placing one of his own patients in the hands of this American caused him to hesitate not one second.

"That seems to me a very good suggestion," he said, as

calmly as he had said everything else that afternoon, so calmly, in fact, that it took me a moment to realize that—wonder of wonders!—he was agreeing unequivocally to my proposal.

We discussed the details. I was on my way to Israel, I told him, but would be returning via London in a month or two. We agreed that by then he would have one or more patients available.

He was as good as his word. Better, in fact, because when he picked me up at my hotel on my return and drove me to the clinic, he had come out into the open.

"I'm so glad that you suggested this," he said, after describing the case I was to operate on. "It shows you are willing to accept any challenge on this. You asked me if I was impressed last time, and I said I was. Well, this is rather more impressive. This is a demonstration of real conviction about stapes mobilization."

At the hospital, he introduced me to his secretary and nurse, gave my instruments to the operating nurse to be sterilized, and cheerfully escorted me to the surgeons' dressing room, where he presented me to half a dozen of his colleagues whom he had alerted. I think it was probable that, if their interest had not already been aroused by a scientific article of mine that had recently appeared, a word from Mr. Cawthorne would have been enough to ensure their presence.

No matter how distinguished a surgeon is, however, he must strip down to his underwear before donning his surgical gown. The dressing or locker room is thus a great leveler. Mr. Cawthorne handed me a gown, and once again I had to admire British simplicity. Instead of the awkward, pajama-like, two-piece affair that American surgeons struggle with daily, it was a simple grayish-blue coverall not unlike the garment mechanics and aviators sometimes wear over their clothing. I had mine on in a jiffy, and we all trooped into the scrub room where I followed the international ritual of all surgeons who intend to approach a patient on the operating table. As I scrubbed my arms, hands, and fingernails for the requisite time, and as I rinsed in antiseptic solution, I could not avoid a small immodesty: the aseptic procedure I was following was one that had been urged on Viennese doctors more than a century before by Semmelweis. He had noticed that childbed fever was a hospital disease and deduced that its cause had something to do with the fact that, in those days, doctors who had come from the deadhouse to the wards never washed or took any precautions against communicating disease from the dead to the living. He begged his colleagues to follow simple aseptic routines. But instead of being acclaimed for his discovery, Semmelweis was scorned, hooted at, hounded, and ultimately driven insane by his colleagues.

There was, let me hasten to add, a large difference between Semmelweis and Rosen—two differences, in fact: Nothing that I have done in medicine can compare in importance with Semmelweis's contribution to the welfare of the world's women and children; and no amount of contempt, abuse, or stupidity could have distracted me from my course at that time. I was no longer in the least doubt about the practicality, safety, and effectiveness of stapes mobilization.

The fact remained, however, that the patient on whom I was about to operate might or might not be one whose hearing stapes mobilization could restore. At that time I was using only the simplest technique: the one that had been so successful in Mr. Lawrence's case; the one that involved only the application of pressure with the mobilizer at the neck of the stapes. As I have said, this was effective in only about one-third of the patients on whom I had tried it, so that there was a real possibility that the woman of about forty chosen by Mr. Cawthorne might have a stapes so encrusted with overgrowth of bone that my mobilizer would fail to budge it.

Too late for these doubts now. The patient lay on the

table, draped and ready for my attentions. Beneath the sterile drapes lay a woman whose welfare had been entrusted confidently to my hands by a brother professional who knew me only by reputation. I had to succeed. And so I got on with it, pausing at each step in the procedure to give each of the gentlemen an opportunity to observe what I had done: the incision around the eardrum, the folding it over on itself to reveal the middle ear, the curetting away of just a bit of the bony canal to obtain a better operative and visual field for the approach to the stapes, and then the attempt to mobilize it.

The mobilizer was in my rubber-gloved hand. "If you will watch my fingers, gentlemen, you will have some concept of the kind of movement I use to exert a kind of rhythmic pressure on the neck of the stapes, so that the stress is exerted through both crura against the footplate." By now, the experience was a familiar one to me, so familiar that I was not the least uncertain when I inserted the mobilizer and guided its tip up the arm of the tiny bone to the point where I could feel through my fingers the notch that meant that the end of the mobilizer lay against the strongest part of the bone. Almost without volition on my part my fingers began the much-practiced movement, gently at first, then more and more powerfully. Quite suddenly, as is often the case, the stapes began to rock under my instrument. The footplate was freed.

"I can hear you now, doctor," the woman's voice came from beneath the drapes. There was a murmur of appreciation and relief among the surgeons and the nurses. "Oh, I can hear all of you really quite well," the patient exclaimed.

"The Lord was with you that time, Sam Rosen," I said to myself. I leaned over the patient and whispered: "Do you like kippers for breakfast?"

"Oh, indeed I do!" she replied.

"What was it you asked her, Sam?" Mr. Cawthorne inquired.

Before I could answer, the patient spoke up: "He asked me if I liked kippers for breakfast, Mr. Cawthorne. Oh, it's really splendid. I can hear you so clearly!"

The drum was soon restored to its normal position, the ear packed, and surgical drapes removed. Everyone in the room was smiling and talking at the same time, the sisters (as senior nurses are called in England), the surgeons, the patient. The most wonderful moments have their element of absurdity. Imagine a room of eight gowned people, seven of them standing and one lying on a table—and all of them grinning idiotically at each other!

Of course the patient was full of gratitude for what had happened. "How can I ever repay you for this, Dr. Rosen?" she asked.

"By being a good patient, and minding what Mr. Cawthorne tells you," I said. "Now, you go back to your bed and we will talk about all this in the morning. It's enough for now that you and I have started something here in London that will spread all over the British Isles."

Until the attendants came, the surgeons talked to her. Imperceptibly they lowered their voices until we were all speaking in almost conspiratorial tones. Then the doors swung open and in came the orderlies, accompanied by several nurses. They were all curious to learn what had happened to this deaf woman. One of them must have slipped out and spread the word, because soon people began entering the operating theatre. Before I knew it there was a score of nurses, orderlies, young doctors, older doctors, all smiling and talking very softly and exchanging comments with the patient. It was, of course, a gross breach of hospital procedure, but no one paid the slightest attention. Something had happened in the past twenty minutes that swept away, for the moment, such considerations.

After the patient had been wheeled away, the doctors and

I went into the dressing room. When we had put on our street clothes, Mr. Cawthorne opened the door and asked one of the nurses if she would be good enough to bring some tea. By his mannered tones, one would have thought that nothing very remarkable had happened, but he obviously wanted to discuss the whole thing right then and there. An impromptu seminar began. Questions and questions, the most thrilling of which to me came from the other doctors: "Could you possibly arrange to come up to Edinburgh (or Manchester, or wherever) and demonstrate this to my people, Dr. Rosen?" As we talked, sometimes seriously, sometimes jestingly—such was our sense of relief that this thing had come off so well— other doctors drifted in, until some had to stand behind those who had found a seat in the dressing room.

As they always had been, they were very gracious, but the atmosphere was now so different. They had seen an event; they had encountered a fact that could not be denied, no matter how many might try to cast doubts upon it. Having seen it, they had to face it, and that meant for many of these men that they had to adjust to a rather overwhelming revolution in their professional lives, for most of them were highly skilled at performing the fenestration operation.

Sometimes when demonstrating stapes mobilization at Mount Sinai, I had had a feeling that the fenestration surgeon watching me would not have been too unhappy if the operation had not succeeded. Who, after all, wants to see years of experience tossed into the discard, a skill painstakingly acquired suddenly rendered as disposable as an empty I.V. bottle? The British are, indeed, a very reserved people. I really had no inkling how those in that dressing room had originally felt, but there was no doubt in my mind that they had accepted what they had seen and were now wholeheartedly on my side. The attitude was revealed in their questions, in their requests that I come to their hospitals and, when the conference finally broke up, in their handshakes.

Handshakes are very revealing. Before the operation, when I had been introduced to these men, we had clasped hands in a friendly sort of way. The grip was moderately firm, but somehow quite formal. The gesture seemed to come more from the brain than from the heart. But now, as they said goodbye, they grabbed my outstretched hand and pumped my arm. We were surgeons, after all, and our hands are totally at the command of our minds, but they almost hurt me in their sudden outrush of feeling toward me.

Finally Mr. Cawthorne and I left the hospital and he put me in a cab to go back to my hotel.

"I've taken the liberty of arranging a little dinner at my club this evening, Dr. Rosen," he said. "I'll call for you at Brown's at seven, if that's convenient."

He had a parcel in his hand that I thought was something he intended to take home, but he handed it to me.

"Now this," he indicated the package. "You've told me that you never accept a fee when you teach abroad, but I thought you would not take it amiss if I gave you one of my surgical gowns. I noticed that you found it very convenient, and I should very much like you to have it."

Of course I accepted both the gift and the invitation. The cab drove off, and on the way to the hotel Sam Rosen, otologist and discoverer of the stapes mobilization, did a very odd thing indeed. He sat back on the cushions and began to cry.

# Of an Opened Door

The dinner at Mr Cawthorne's club was as pleasant as one could imagine. The next day I went to another hospital in London and, my lucky star still being ascendant, went through the performance successfully with another British surgeon's patient. Then it was time to return to New York and be once more the prophet at home.

After a while, however, the waves that crossed the Atlantic in both directions began to meet and stir up a fair amount of foam. From the western shore they carried the message, "We don't think much of Rosen or his work," but from the opposite side came waves of opinion that said, "Some of us have seen what he does, and we think we ought to give it a try before we condemn it."

In a few years the conflict that raged among my colleagues—and within them as well—slowly worked itself out. Who was this Rosen who was upsetting their nicely ordered way of life? A Harvard or a Johns Hopkins man? A gentleman among gentlemen? Not a bit of it. Perhaps he wasn't, like Julius

Lempert, the graduate of a diploma mill, but, well, his M.D. from Syracuse in 1921 hardly distinguished him. Yet he was an associate of Friesner, an attending at Mount Sinai, and everybody knew Sam Rosen. Not a bad fellow, really, except for his association with people like Henry Wallace. And on the other hand there was the insistent logic of Rosen's operation. After all, damn it, it worked, if not invariably, then often enough so that a man really should try mobilization before subjecting a patient to fenestration with all that that entailed.

It seemed almost without warning that I found myself receiving some of the top men in my specialty. Could they observe a mobilization? Yes, of course. They came, one by one; they watched; they listened; they went the Bellevue route and performed cadaver operations under my direction. These were not little-known but devoted men from obscure parts of the country. They were leaders in otology, and they returned to their medical centers where they followed my injunction to practice, practice, practice on cadavers before attempting to operate on a living patient.

Before I knew it, at medical meetings I would find myself surrounded by eight or ten surgeons asking me questions about this or that aspect of the mobilization procedure: What kinds of patients were good prospects for it? What techniques did I use to cope with this or that situation?

"Well, in that situation," I would perhaps say, "it might be advisable to use a slightly different instrument that I've worked out. You can go down to the footplate with this and make perforations to loosen it up a little."

"Is that safe? Isn't that likely to cause labyrinthitis?"

"I haven't published my results yet, but so far I haven't encountered any untoward effects," I would answer.

Well, now, how could they get one of these new perforators? And should they practice with it on the cadaver and on temporal bone specimens?

Of course they should, I said, explaining that naturally I

had done many such operations before trying it on patients. Several companies were now making sets of instruments according to my designs. As for temporal bones, I had a splendid source of supply by then. I had been to Germany and Austria, where the mores regarding autopsies are very different from ours. It occurred to me that some of the dieners there might not be averse to learning how to remove the temporal bones of the skull in a way which left the deceased's appearance quite intact. The trick was to approach the bone, and the inner and middle ear structures that it contained, from inside the skull. Inspired by the thought of extra income, the European dieners soon learned how to do this, and obligingly supplied me with hundreds of specimens preserved in formalin. When these arrived at customs offices in this country, conspicuously labeled "Anatomical Specimens—Human," our American way of looking at death proved very useful. They were passed without inspection.

In no time at all, I miraculously changed from an otological version of the "invisible man" to a great pal of my colleagues. Dr. Rosen vanished in favor of good old Sam. It was "Hey there, Sam," and "Gee, that's great, Sam," and "What's the latest on mobilizations, Sam?" and Sam this and Sam that. It was as if suddenly the whole world of my specialty was lit up with Roman candles and other fireworks proclaiming what a great fellow this Sam Rosen with his stapes mobilization was.

And I enjoyed every delicious moment of it. Of course I did. The years of being sneered at, of being ignored, doubted, even reviled were over. It was a great satisfaction to walk through the hotel corridors like that lion in the mutual fund ads on television who strides powerfully out of the subway station and down Wall Street. In the TV commercial, passers-by never seem to notice the lion, no doubt because it is a trick shot in which the lion is somehow photographed against a moving backdrop of an ordinary street scene. He isn't really there. He is as invisible to the passers-by as I had been for so many years. But now I was very much the real lion. Oh, it was a delight and a joy, and I tried to exult in it as unnoticeably as human nature would allow, but many a night in sheer pleasure I couldn't resist phoning Helen back in New York to tell her about how some particularly pompous member of my profession had cornered me that day to demonstrate to our colleagues what great friends he and I had been all along, and how intimate his knowledge was of stapes mobilization, and how, all along, he had been one of the strongest proponents of the new surgery— and by the way, would I be able to come out to Megalopolis Medical Center next month and do, uh, two or three demonstration operations on some of his patients, not that *he* needed the instruction so much as some of the younger men on his staff and others in Megalopolis who hadn't pioneered in this work like us . . . Such little dramas gave me many a secret laugh, and Helen and me later a good, loud, hearty guffaw.

There was still one more hurdle that had to be leaped. That was to arrange to present the accumulated results of my work before the Supreme Court of the otological world, the American Laryngological, Rhinological and Otological Society, known mercifully for short as the "Triological." Some members of this society are as lugubriously self-important as the name sounds, but in fairness it has to be said also that others are as straight and to the point as its nickname.

What I had to report was no longer speculative. The results had been measured over a broad enough spectrum of cases and a sufficient length of time so that there could no longer be any doubt about the matter: stapes mobilization was effective in a certain percentage of cases. But my purpose in presenting this material to the Triological was not just to put it on the record and—not incidentally—to give it the imprimatur of this most important body. I wanted to stir up everybody in the field, get them thinking about mobilization, get them working to improve on it. No therapeutic procedure works in every case, but I knew that if my colleagues, especially the younger, less hidebound ones, would go after it, they would find all sorts of ways to improve on it, to make it work better, and to make it work in cases where it still failed. I was sure that some of them would overtake and pass me in devising ingenious ways to overcome some of the problems that still prevented the restoration of hearing to men and women who were theoretically perfectly acceptable candidates for the procedure. Every sensible person anticipates such development of a new technique or of any discovery.

Far from shrinking from the thought of improvements being made on the operation, I had begun sometime earlier to try to improve on it myself. The original procedure worked well, but it worked well in only about one-third of the cases. What to do about the others?

What to do? Why, back to the instrument maker and the deadhouse, of course. The Grafraths enthusiastically supplied me with several variations of a long, needle-sharp probe. With the right one, depending upon the exact anatomy of the particular cadaver ear I was trying it on, I could make tiny perforations around the rim of the footplate. After much practice, I tried the technique on a patient whose stapes could not be freed no matter how much pressure I exerted at the stapes neck. Carefully, so as not to enter the inner ear, I made minute holes around the border of the footplate with the new instrument and then tried to mobilize the bone in the usual way. It came free. Here was a case that, until then, would have had to be assigned for a fenestration but which would now not require that difficult procedure.

Working in this way, and teaching the few otologists who had sought me out, I soon accumulated more than two hundred cases. On each, Dr. Bergman and I had developed as precise information as was humanly possible. Sooner or later, the

Triological powers-that-be would want to hear Rosen, and that would be the occasion for presenting the most scientifically accurate information. To do the best possible job, we had to take careful measurements of the ability of each patient to hear pure tones in each ear, both before and after the operation, and then follow up on each one for as long as possible. In addition, wherever possible, we measured the speech reception thresholds of each patient's ears, because the ability to understand speech is even more important to the patient than the purely diagnostic and predictive information provided by testing his ability to hear pure tones at various frequencies. Finally, there was the ever-present question of how to treat the statistics. What constituted a success, what a failure? To be strictly scientific about our data, we decided to treat every single patient that we were not able to follow up month after month after the operation as failures. They might be hearing superbly, but we had no way of knowing that. Some researchers "solve" this problem by simply dropping these patients out of the total number entirely, but to do this is to hedge on one's results. It distorts the picture of the overall results because it does not picture the true percentage of success in a series of cases.

We were ready when, at last, a letter came from Dr. Stewart Nash, secretary of the Triological, inviting me to present a paper on stapes mobilization. The meeting was to be held in Hollywood, Florida, in 1955. It was wintertime. Physicians always manage to arrange to meet in Florida or Puerto Rico in the winter, and in cooler climes during the summer.

I showed the letter to my secretary, Mrs. Belle Sien, and called Helen to tell her the news. Both of them would have to come with me to Hollywood. They had been through all of it with me, the very bad times, the merely bad times, and now the good ones, and they were entitled to see what was in the pot at the end of the rainbow. It was exciting, even if it was inevitable. As soon as Belle had typed my letter of acceptance,

I signed it and ran out onto Park Avenue to mail it myself. From that moment I felt like a different man. For the first time, most of the really top men in my specialty would be present to listen to my paper, to evaluate my technique, to scrutinize my statistical results. A few had already been to see me, had watched me operate, and had gone away to practice on cadavers and try the operation on patients. Now the most skilled and the most prestigious men in the specialty would have to come to grips with this once and for all.

The meeting lasted three or four days, during each of which there were four- or five-hour sessions in which men from all over the United States and Canada read papers and discussed them. To my dismay, I discovered that I was scheduled to deliver the very last paper of the meeting. When I asked Dr. Nash the reason for this, he said: "Well, Sam, it's stirred up a storm. I believe in you, and I know you've got something valuable here. Some others don't; you know that. But they can't wait to hear you, just the same. So the program committee decided the way to keep them all here for the entire meeting was to make them wait for the Rosen paper until the end!"

Naturally, this was both pleasing and irritating. It was hard to listen patiently to the papers presented by others, some of which were excellent and some less than earth-shaking in their import. It was good to have Helen and Belle there. They had not only been through it all; they had carefully edited and typed and re-edited and retyped the papers I had already written. This one was the same. We had gone over it again and again, but now I insisted that we examine every last word once more. Was there a sentence that should go in here? Should this come out? Was this overstated? Should this other thing be emphasized a little more and that played down a little bit? No mother with her first baby was ever fussier. You know what I mean: if the baby cries, something terrible is wrong; and if the baby *doesn't* cry, why, there must also be something the matter with it! I fussed and fussed, and Belle retyped and retyped. She must have made a dozen revisions during those few days, but finally I ran out of nits to pick and the paper was there, ready for delivery, final, irrevocable—and still there was a day to wait before delivering it.

That day ground slowly on toward the appointed hour. As the next to last speaker read his presentation, the ballroom slowly filled, until there were physicians and surgeons standing along the walls. Men from all over the world were assembled and in a few minutes Sam Rosen from Syracuse would have to show his infant to the cold, cold world. The speaker concluded. A few men came to the platform and discussed it briefly. The speaker answered them. Then the chairman took the microphone . . .

It would not be accurate to say that my heart was in my mouth as he introduced me. It was somewhere down in my shoes. As I walked up the aisle to take the microphone, it felt as though I were walking through icy mud. It was not the first time I had delivered a scientific paper, but never had so much attention been focused on me before.

"You have the facts, Sam," I kept saying to myself as I approached the podium. "Don't worry about any of it; don't worry about criticism, because that's the way it ought to be. And don't worry about hostility and opposition, because no matter how big the gun that's shooting at you, the shells are going to be made of opinions, while yours are made of tough, hard, armor-piercing facts."

Twenty minutes, during which I read, slowly, carefully, putting on slides to show the stages of the operation, representative before-and-after audiograms, and tables of statistical results. Twenty minutes, and then, after a moment of silence, tremendous applause. They were all clapping. Looking out at them as the lights went up, I realized suddenly that the turning point had come. There would be discussion, criticism, comment, argument, but the main thing had already happened: my colleagues were finally convinced. They finally had come to the conviction that Rosen's mobilization was an authentic discovery in the treatment of conductive deafness.

As the discussants made their points, it became clear that they were no longer as hostile as I had expected them to be. A vigorous defense was legitimate, but I was careful not to make it personal. Every criticism I answered, often conceding that there remained more to be done with this new operation.

"It's only the beginning," I told them. "The door has been opened, that's all. Now we must all go through that door and see what's in the room on the other side."

# Of Prejudice

---

Beyond that door there turned out to be not one but many rooms. From an operation capable of curing only about one-third of the patients suffering from otosclerosis, stapes mobilization has been developed into a series of techniques, each adapted to the particular conditions a surgeon may encounter, so that today the cure rate at the hands of a highly skilled operator is as high as 80 to 90 per cent. Here and there I have been privileged to add important items of furniture to those rooms, but my colleagues all over the world, and especially in this country, have made invaluable contributions.

A lot of detail would probably be boring, but some of the more ingenious techniques ought to be mentioned. In California, for instance, Dr. Howard House decided that when the crura of the stapes broke off during an attempted mobilization, one should not give up. Instead he cut them off entirely, leaving the rigid footplate in the oval window. Then, with a needle-pointed probe, he broke the footplate in many places, creating

**169**

a comminuted fracture of the remaining bone. From the incus, he suspended a small strut of polyethylene which he deftly cut to just the right length so that it touched the fractured plate of bone, forming an artificial stapes to replace the missing crura. This marvelous technique worked so well that it raised the percentage of successful operations markedly—from about 35 to 60 per cent.

There were others who devised techniques to deal with further problems. One of these was Dr. John Shea. A vigorous, alert young surgeon, he came up from Memphis soon after the Florida meeting to study the original technique at Mount Sinai, watching one operation after another, and working steadily with me on cadavers at Bellevue. It was impossible to give him enough experience in a short time, so I urged him to go to Vienna where I had demonstrated the procedure and had learned that there was a really adequate supply of cadavers. John took my advice. In a short time he returned, having performed some two hundred cadaver operations. Returning to Memphis, he began to do the original operation with the same success rate as mine. Then, when Dr. House announced his improvement, he began using that technique. Finally, he developed the concept of stapedectomy: of taking out the stapes entirely, covering the oval window with a piece of vein, and installing a prosthetic stapes of tungsten wire or polyethylene (see Figure 4C p. 124). It worked very well; it simplified the whole operation, because one did not have to make tricky judgments about each case in the middle of the operation. But in the course of time it developed that a few of these radically treated patients lost their hearing completely, probably because of the extremes of manipulation and because the irritation induced by putting in foreign tissue right at the opening to the inner ear causes inflammation and damage to the nerve of hearing. In other cases, there seemed to be leakage of the inner-ear fluid, the perilymph, causing loss of wave motion within or nerve damage, or both.

Nevertheless, stapedectomy has proved of value. We have learned how to use a synthetic material called Gelfoam together with a prosthesis made of wire and Teflon in cases where removing the stapes entirely is the only way in which hearing can be restored. The combination usually results in the formation of a thin, flexible membrane across the opening of the oval window—a new, natural windowpane which holds in the perilymph but vibrates with the prosthetic stapes to conduct sound waves to the fluid and thence to the delicate apparatus of the nerve of hearing.

What a hectic period the year following that Triological meeting was! Science writers attending the meeting besieged me. One was Roland Berg, science editor of *Look*. He had interviewed me in New York, had watched the surgery performed, had talked to patients. In due course an article in *Look* appeared, by William Chapman White, entitled "New Hope for the Deaf." The effect was to galvanize the public. Patients began to besiege their otologists. They wanted the Rosen operation, and they wanted it *now*. Surgeons who had been reluctant to take up mobilization had to face the fact that, if they did not learn the technique, their patients would surely go to someone else, either at home, or in some other city. If I had ever doubted the power of the press I doubted it no more. It seems that there is nothing so effective as an informed patient when it comes to mobilizing a whole profession into action.

Now there was no lack, either of patients or of eager students. They came from all points of the compass, and since there was an unending stream of good candidates for the operation, it was always possible to teach the operation to groups of five or six visiting surgeons, after which we would go to Bellevue for additional direct, practical experience on the dead. Not one qualified man was turned away, and sometimes a surgeon from a remote part of the country would find himself working side by side with the most distinguished men in our specialty.

An innovation can evidently be a great equalizer. Before

it is accepted, the lowliest carper is listened to by the great and
near-great with respect. Afterward, however, all are suddenly
on the same bare ground, clean slates ready to be written upon
with such words of wisdom as a man can summon up at such
a moment. It does take time for a new idea to gain acceptance.
"This time," Dr. John Stokes of University College Hospital in
London has observed,

> like the ages of man, can be divided into seven phases . . . :
> (1) I don't believe it (2) It won't work (3) The numbers are
> not statistically significant (4) It's dangerous (5) It's not pos-
> sible to make it generally available, and then, after a little while:
> (6) Of course, we've known it all the time and (7) Actually
> we thought of it first ourselves.

Dr. Stokes had good English precedent for this observation.
The great seventeenth-century physician and naturalist William
Harvey had just such an experience. According to Sir William
Osler, Harvey waited twelve years, during each of which he
demonstrated his discovery of the circulation of the blood to all
comers, "before daring to publish the facts on which the truth
was based." In his revolutionary monograph on the subject,
*Exercitatio anatomica de motu cordis et sanguinis in animalibus,*
published in 1628, Harvey wrote: "These views, as usual pleased
some more, others less; some chid and calumniated me, and
laid it to me as a crime that I had dared to depart from the
precepts and opinions of all Anatomists."

Of course, no responsible researcher expects his colleagues
to take anything new for granted. They rightly want proof of
the pudding, and especially do they want it in the form of what
Dr. Stokes refers to as "the numbers." One successful operation
does not make a cure, but several hundred are another matter,
especially when all are carefully presented—successes, partial
successes, outright failures, and cases lost to follow-up.

My own experience with those who "chid and calumniated" would have infuriated a saint. For three years my colleagues had turned a deaf ear to my entreaties to come and see the operation, look at, question and test the patients, examine the results, and learn how to go and do likewise. It all happened years ago, but when a man sits down to write a memoir, he thinks over the whole of the past. He wonders if he can somehow make it all whole, if he can bring it all together into a comprehensible pattern, like a model diagnosis. Why this massive reluctance to accept what was obviously inevitable? Certainly the attempt to ignore and ostracize me went far beyond the proper scientific skepticism of reasonable men. What crime, then, had I committed?

There were several. My "no reprints" colleague came to me finally, for example, and made his peace. We had had a "misunderstanding," he said. I let it go at that, partly because I was eager to see this thing spread far and wide for the benefit of deaf people everywhere. In reality, however, there was no misunderstanding. He and most of the others understood very well that here was something new that threatened to render obsolete a skill they had painstakingly acquired, often at great expense, and now practiced in return for handsome financial rewards and professional and lay esteem. To do a complicated, delicate four-hour surgical procedure makes one a hero, and a wealthy hero at that.

Thinking about it recently, it suddenly dawned on me that this aspect of the reasons for such determined opposition had been subtly confirmed to me by one of America's greatest ear surgeons. I tend to be rather blunt of speech, I guess, and it apparently works two ways: little hints don't make much of an impression upon me. In this case, the hint came when the surgeon in question was visiting me at my home in Westchester. We sat on the porch, talking shop, of course.

"Sam, you've told me about that first mobilization," my

colleague said. "What I don't quite understand is, what caused you to jump to the conclusion that you had found a new way to treat otosclerosis?"

The question amazed me. Why, wasn't it obvious that, if the patient could suddenly hear as a result of my mobilizing his stapes, here was a whole new world to explore? I said as much, and added: "What would you have done in my place?"

"Well, to tell the truth," he said casually, "I think I might have just gone right on doing fenestrations."

He was not the only one who asked me what had caused me to investigate stapes mobilization. Each time I gave what seemed to me to be the obvious answer, and almost as often the questioner shook his head in wonder, seeming to say that to ignore what I had experienced would have been a far more natural reaction.

Money and politics. They were sufficient motive powers to produce the fierce opposition—or were they? No, there was another possibility that finally occurred to me. I am a Jew, and ours is a racist country, sad to say. Medicine is tainted with this disease just as are the other professions. As part of the research for this book, I looked up a number of people who knew me in those days and who were in a position, possibly, to know what was really going on. One of them was a science writer who had followed my work closely from the moment that word of it first appeared in the *New York State Journal of Medicine*.

He had become convinced, after watching me operate and examining my records, that stapes mobilization was something important. But as a real "pro," he checked with the experts—or people he had a right to believe were experts: that is, the leading otologists in the country. What did they think of the Rosen operation? he asked. This question was met with bland assertions that they knew next to nothing of my work, but the journalist knew his business and was prepared for that. He produced reprints of my journal articles and offered to update them with information he had gathered directly from me since their publication. The experts waved the papers away. Well, yes, they *had* heard of it, of course, but there was really nothing to it; Rosen's notion was contrary to all sound otological principles, and besides fenestration was reliable, predictable, and usually effective.

That did not satisfy my journalist friend. He had no inhibitions about looking more deeply into the matter. He wondered out loud why Dr. Rosen had not been invited to present his results at the annual meetings of the Triological? The answers were even more evasive, if possible: How did he know Rosen hadn't been invited? (As if Rosen would turn down such an invitation!) What business was it of his whom the specialty chose to invite to present papers at its meetings? Would the journalist please excuse the specialist now, since he had patients to see and other urgent matters to attend to?

His suspicions thoroughly aroused, the journalist went to see a prominent otologist and put the case bluntly.

"I've read Dr. Rosen's case studies and his papers," he said, "and it's obvious that he has something here of tremendous importance to your specialty. There are thousands, maybe millions of people in this country alone who might benefit from this operation, if only the otologists learned how to do it."

"There's nothing to stop them," my colleague said coldly.

"Oh, but there is!" the journalist said. "You know as well as I do that the Triological has to sprinkle holy water on it before a lot of otologists will even consider it. It has to have the sanction of the society, but Dr. Rosen tells me he gets the cold shoulder every time he tries to arrange to deliver a paper. Now, I know that Dr. Rosen isn't exactly conventional. No doubt he's been a thorn in the side of a lot of his—"

"He certainly has," my colleague burst out angrily. "He's been nothing but a troublemaker. He's the kind that has always gotten the Jews into deep trouble throughout history, and as far as I am concerned, I hope he never gets a chance to present any so-called results of his so-called mobilization operation to the Triological!"

From that office, the journalist went to the elegant consulting room of a leading member of the Triological. Here, he told me, he got the same reception and was told the same story, although in more refined, Anglo-Saxon accents.

"Well, you see, Mr. ____," the great man said smoothly, "we in the society feel that Dr. Rosen is, ah, rather unreliable. You know his reputation and his, ah, background. Even some of his closest associates have suggested that it might not be best for the specialty to give too much credence to his claims. At the very least it would be premature. At best it might result in a great deal of disappointment to the thousands of patients who, as you say, suffer from conductive hearing loss."

My usually good-natured journalist friend was really outraged at this, he told me years later. Instead of going away quietly, he threatened to bring the whole sordid story out into the open, and he had the power to do this, since he had access to the media on a national level. Then he went away, and shortly thereafter, it seems, came the invitation to present my results at the next meeting of the Triological.

Perhaps that was just a coincidence. Perhaps the tight little band of men who nominate each other to high office in the society had decided just about then that the time had come to give me my day in otology's Supreme Court. There is no way to tell, and I am sure that my colleagues in the society will resent my recounting with "typical Jewish ingratitude" this seamy tale. But racism, if that is what it was, is one of the world's most deadly diseases. In Hitler's time, it caused the death of millions, directly in the case of the Jews who were exterminated, indirectly in the case of others of all nationalities, including Germans, who were killed during World War II. I loathe and fear it, but I will not be silent about racism in any form, be it anti-Semitism, discrimination against blacks or Orientals, or racist attitudes on the part of blacks toward whites, or any other kind.

Furthermore, I won't practice it. Over the past two decades, I have traveled from one country to another teaching what I have learned. When some of my friends learned that I had agreed to go to Egypt and to Jordan to teach, they were scandalized. How could a good Jew do such a thing? How could I contemplate consorting with the sworn enemies of Israel? Later, when friends learned that I had agreed to go to Spain for the same purpose they were equally shocked. How could I, a man of leftist convictions, set foot in a Fascist country created by Hitler, Mussolini, and Franco on the murdered corpse of the Republic of Spain?

I could and did. My Jewish heritage and my political convictions teach me to put humanity before every other consideration. Why, even today I operate and teach in a country that is conducting history's most insane and inhumane war—in Indochina. Should I put down my scalpel and refuse to help deaf Americans on that account? Should I self-righteously decline to teach American ear surgeons because perhaps the majority of them have supported this hideous war in Vietnam?

Long ago I decided that any patient and any surgeon who could benefit by my knowledge and skill would get the best that I could provide. One American surgeon once asked me to come to his city to demonstrate the operation to him and his colleagues. I accepted, of course, even though I know him to be notoriously and offensively anti-Semitic. Imagine my surprise when he invited me to dinner at his home, a gesture that was roughly equivalent to Governor George Wallace inviting Mrs. Martin Luther King. Imagine his relief when I declined. Later, after I returned from that expedition to middle America, a colleague—not a Jew, but not an anti-Semite either—told me how enormously relieved that man had been that I had not accepted his hospitality. He might have been less pleased had he known that under no circumstance, except on a medical call, would I set foot in the home of such a man.

During the Middle Ages, according to the historian of medicine Dr. Henry E. Sigerist, Christians were forbidden, on pain of excommunication, to call in non-Christian physicians. "The superiority of the Arabic and Jewish physicians, however, was so evident," Dr. Sigerist wrote,* "that it was impossible to enforce this rule." There seems to be a lesson here somewhere.

It would be unfair to end this chapter on such a note. No body of men is without its pettifoggers, its charlatans, its men of ill will. Nor, in my experience, is any man free of the glories and the taints of his time. The American, black or white, doesn't breathe who doesn't somewhere harbor in him a secret sense of superiority to "gooks" of whatever foreign nationality. There is some of the saint and some of the sinner in every one of us, and this goes for the members of my profession too. Most are dedicated men, and most possess more than a fair share of smugness and overweening pride in their accomplishments, their splendid lives of service to their patients, and their general superiority to the common ruck of mankind. And while it may be that I have developed some antibodies to these diseases of the human mind, I make no claim to total immunity. All I ask is to be seen for what I am—an ordinary human being—and to be forgiven for that. One of the nicest compliments ever paid me was by a neighbor who works by the hour mowing lawns and clipping hedges. One day during the worst of the Fearful Fifties, someone remarked to him that that Dr. Rosen was a Communist.

"Oh, yes," the man replied, according to a friend who later told me about the conversation. "That Dr. Rosen is a mighty fine man. You'd never think he was one of those Park Avenue doctors: he's just as common as anybody."

* In *On the History of Medicine* (New York: MD Publications, 1960).

# Of a Magic Carpet

Some people who have read the foregoing description of the resistance and hostility to stapes mobilization have commented that it seems exaggerated. It is hard to know where to draw the line in describing a phenomenon like this. I don't want to be unfair, or give the wrong impression. Certainly every scientist has the right, even the duty, to maintain a high index of skepticism whenever he looks at something new. On the other hand, there is all too much truth to the statement of Britain's Dr. John Stokes, cited before, that for a new idea to gain acceptance a progression ranging from absolute incredulity to self-appropriation must take place. In like vein, more than half a century of experience in medicine has led Dr. Walter C. Alvarez, editor emeritus of *Modern Medicine*, to observe:

> First, for many years the innovator's work is ignored and no man will mention or quote it. Then, if forced to admit that they have heard of his work, several men will say, "There is nothing

to it; he is all wrong." And finally when many men are talking about the work and praising it, the detractors will say, "Oh, that was nothing; it was known long before and was discovered by a man in Vienna."

That has been my experience, with certain added overtones and undertones. Now, however, let's be done with it and move on to other things.

Moving on was just what I did, too. Helen, that indomitable spirit, had already started the process early in the 1950's. As a young woman, she had traveled a great deal, but since our marriage, we stayed close to home. At first it was to build my practice; then it was the children; then it was the war; then it was the Progressive Party and Henry Wallace.

By 1951 (before my encounter with Mr. Lawrence's stapes), the reason could very well have become the fact that my practice was in a shambles and ought to be painstakingly rebuilt. We could have stayed home in order to lick our wounds and recover from the blows, but Helen wanted to be off and doing things. Not I, though. The lure of my "vine and fig tree" in Katonah was powerful. Who needed to go dashing about all over Europe? Every summer we had guests over for tennis and swimming, for cook-outs and conversation. What could Europe offer that could be better than a leisurely summer in Katonah? Besides, we couldn't afford it.

Helen knew how to deal with these objections. She ignored some, but advanced counter-arguments as well. Then Jo and Florence Davidson wrote inviting us to stay with them in the south of France. This was followed by an invitation to me to lecture at the school of medicine at Tours. Not too long after these seemingly unrelated events, Helen calmly announced that she had rented our Katonah place lock, stock, and tennis ball for the summer. The rent money would cover the costs of a trip to Europe for the four of us if we were careful. Furthermore, she told me, a four-bunk cabin on the *Queen Mary* had already been booked. It was obvious that Helen, John, Judy, and I were bound for Europe that summer.

It was such a relief to get away from the United States and its hysteria. We laughed and giggled our way across the Atlantic, drawing lots each night to see who would sleep in the two upper bunks in the cabin. When Helen drew one, the three of us would pretend that she couldn't make it and go about laboriously hoisting her bodily into the bunk.

On the train from Le Havre there was more hilarity. Helen and the children, who were then nineteen and sixteen, knew some French, but I had nary a word. On the way to Paris they decided to teach me numbers, reciting "Un, deux, trois, quatre . . ." over and over again, and having me repeat after them. We were as quiet as possible so as not to disturb the other passengers. They got me up to "six" but somehow I couldn't remember "sept" to save my soul. I went back to "Un" to get a running start, but it was no use. "Sept" would not come to my lips. I paused and at least half the passengers in the car looked over their newspapers and cried in unison: "sept!"

Fortunately, the street number of the tiny hotel we stayed at in Paris was "quatre." Each time I left it alone, Judy and John would take me aside and have me repeat "quatre, Boulevard Raspail, quatre, Boulevard Raspail, quatre, Boulevard Raspail," until they were satisfied that taxi drivers and gendarmes would be able to return me safely if I got lost.

After the Tours lecture, it was time for me to fly to Israel, where I had other teaching engagements. Helen and the children would drive through France to Rome where I was to meet them later. On the flight to Tel Aviv I had time to think, time to recall how reluctant I had been to take this trip at all. Thank heaven that Helen had brushed aside my objections! It was my first time abroad and here I was fifty-four years old. It occurred to me that I had been in real danger of slipping into a comfortable, middle-aged rut that I might have followed without thinking for the rest of my life. It was a narrow escape.

The Israeli health authorities had asked me to lecture on Ménière's disease and to demonstrate my procedure for sectioning the chorda tympani as a preliminary surgical procedure that I believe is useful in treating this often crippling condition. The victim of Ménière's disease suffers from severe vertigo, nausea, vomiting, the sensation of noise in the affected ear, and deafness. The disease is fickle. Attacks come without warning, last for days or weeks, and then subside, if the patient is lucky. During an attack, the patient often cannot walk because his equilibrium is completely destroyed. His misery is so great that some patients admit that their real fear is that they are *not* going to die from it.

Medical treatment is always tried first, as it should be. If all else fails, the surgeon is brought in and asked to destroy, either by the use of ultrasonic waves or by physical obliteration, the nerves that lie within the semicircular canal on that side. Unfortunately, this drastic procedure often destroys the nerve of hearing which is so intimately associated with the nerve of equilibrium.

The chorda tympani passes through the middle ear. When I was regularly performing Lempert's fenestrations, I tried cutting the chorda and using it as a graft to keep the newly made fenestra from closing over. It seemed to me that the patients in whom I tried this technique suffered from much less vertigo following the operation than those in whom vein grafts were made. Could there be some connection between the chorda and the vestibular nerve, the nerve of equilibrium? Reviewing the literature led me to Dr. Laurenti de No, the famed neurohistologist and neuroanatomist at The Rockefeller University. Dr. de No confirmed that his studies showed that the chorda, as it continued on its course upward from the middle ear to the brain, not only lay adjacent to the vestibular nerve but was literally connected to it by several small nerve fibers.

By 1951, I had done about a hundred chorda tympani sections as a treatment for Ménière's disease, using the same surgical approach—Lempert's tympano-sympathectomy incision—as I later used for stapes mobilization. In three out of four cases, the procedure seemed to relieve the patient. This result sounds better than it really is. Ménière's, as I have said, often goes into remission of its own accord, so that it is impossible to say that the operation produced favorable results in 75 per cent of the cases. It is only possible to say that it failed to produce such a result in 25 per cent.

Under the circumstances, it was easy to understand why no one, so far as I know, has adopted the operation. On a second look, however, one might wonder why surgeons who treat Ménière's disease by labyrinthectomy have not tried chorda tympani section first. It's such an innocuous procedure. It takes no more than ten or fifteen minutes under local anesthesia. One reflects the drum in the way I have already described, cuts through the nerve, and then replaces the drum. The patient need not be hospitalized more than a few hours. In view of this, perhaps it is not logical to proceed directly from medical treatment to the most drastic of surgical procedures for Ménière's disease: the obliteration of the whole labyrinth and its nerve of equilibrium.

The Israeli health authorities shared this view to some extent, and invited me to come and teach their ear surgeons how to do it. At Lydda Airport, outside Tel Aviv, I was met by the Israeli Health Minister, Dr. Chaim Sheba, two or three other doctors, and Yan Yanai of the Foreign Ministry. They had a limousine waiting to take me to Tel Aviv, but as we started to drive away I saw something that made me ask the driver to stop a moment.

The car stopped near an old Dakota, or DC-3, from which a

stream of unkempt people were emerging, carrying what were obviously their only possessions. They looked exhausted, but as soon as they reached the ground, they stooped and kissed it and burst into tears. It was hard not to do the same.

"They are Yemenite Jews," one of my companions offered. He explained that Israel had arranged with all Arab countries to bring any Jews who wanted to come to Israel, regardless of age, health, or wealth. This group was obviously of every age from babe in arms to bearded patriarch, and in every state of health. Of wealth they had none. The Israelis were running daily flights to any land where there were Jewish refugees in order to bring them home. The flights were called "the magic carpet," and when you looked at the mass of people that the tired old Dakota had carried, you believed that some magic was surely involved.

As I operated and taught during the next days, I kept thinking of that scene. I wanted to go on one of those flights. I wanted to be a part of this, see what it was all about. When I expressed my interest to various officials, they shook their heads. It was dangerous. If the flight were to an Arab country and the government should find out that I had illicitly participated in such a flight, there would be all kinds of trouble, mostly for me. I would find myself a Jew in an Arab country without a proper visa and without protection.

I tried to content myself with seeing the country, talking with otologists and health ministry people, and teaching what I knew about Ménière's disease and its treatment. Everywhere there were signs of a young nation being built despite tremendous difficulties. As we drove to the Hadassah Hospital in Tel Aviv one morning, my escort, one of the otologists there, took a new route. New buildings were going up everywhere.

"It was just a desert a few years ago," he told me, "and the people who live in these new apartments were living in *marborats.*"

I knew that meant the shanty towns that one still saw

everywhere, and the thought intruded that those Yemenites were already probably living in *marborats* somewhere in Tel Aviv. Yet the government and the people welcomed them, the old and sick, the young and vigorous. I don't believe that in the history of mankind there has been so large an in-migration in so short a time to such a tiny country.

After I had been in Israel about a week, I woke up one morning feeling strangely different. At first, I could not identify the new feeling. I felt marvelously relaxed. I was happy in a way I had never felt before. As usual I got up, breakfasted, was driven to the hospital. As I worked, I thought about how I felt, and gradually it dawned on me that for the first time I was in an environment free of anti-Semitism. At last I knew what it was to live where there was no undercurrent of race or ethnic prejudice. Everyone was busy building not only his own future but the future of his fellow men. This was what the American pioneers must have felt. This was the taste of freedom.

Since that first trip, Helen and I have been to Israel several times. We have watched the country grow and prosper, despite the hostility of the Arab countries all around it, with pride and elation. We have also, sad to say, seen what has happened as Israel turned toward industrialization, became more and more dependent on foreign, mostly U.S. capital, and involved itself more and more deeply in the big power politics of the Middle East confrontation between the United States and the U.S.S.R. Much of the vigorous, young pioneering spirit has now disappeared. The emphasis on communal living in the rural kibbutzim has given way to a search for individual self-aggrandizement. I don't pretend to know the answers, but I wonder where it will all end. I wonder how wise the Israelis are to put most of their trust in the United States which, like all governments, can only be counted on to act in its own interests —or rather, what its leaders rightly or mistakenly conceive to be its interests.

On that first visit, however, no such misgivings assailed me.

One of my patients was an Arab sheik, an important and wealthy resident of Nazareth, and an Israeli citizen. He was about forty-five and had been having frequent bouts of vertigo, tinnitus (noise in the ear), and the other classic signs of Ménière's disease. It was only a matter of minutes to perform the chorda tympani section on the affected ear. The next day he returned to Nazareth, and I went on with my work, thinking no more about it.

Near the end of my stay, however, the sheik appeared at my hotel with his wife, a beautiful young woman with black hair, dark brown eyes, and a full, round figure.

"My husband does not speak English," she said gravely, "and so he brought me along to thank you so much for what you have done. He has not had an attack of dizziness or nausea since the operation five weeks ago."

"It was kind of you to come all this way to tell me about it," I said.

"Oh, it is not so far by motor car," she said, "and besides, my husband wants me to say that we would be honored if you and as many of your colleagues as you would care to bring would come to our home in Nazareth. We want to celebrate the occasion with a feast."

When I went to the hospital the next day, I mentioned this to the doctors. They were enthusiastic. The sheik's table would not be rationed, unlike their own.

"Meat!" one of them exclaimed. "I don't remember when I have tasted meat."

It was arranged. Early the next afternoon three cars filled with otologists and other physicians drove through the soft green hills to Nazareth. As the sun set, we drove up to the minarets of Nazareth, set like a jewel on a high point of ground.

The sheik and his wife greeted us at the entrance to their large stone house and escorted us inside to meet their friends who had assembled for the feast. As darkness fell, we sat down to a long, narrow table on which stood a huge, steaming, food-filled cauldron. Dinner was gay and bountiful. Shy, young Arab girls, their bare feet caked with dirt, served us lamb, rice, vegetables, and fruits. From where I sat, I could look out the window at the stars, hanging like distant lamps in the silent sky. I wondered if Helen was also looking at that star that moment. I wondered what she would say if she knew I was dining in an Arab home in the middle of Israel. And I wondered whether somewhere in some arid Arab land, another group of immigrants was waiting for "the magic carpet" to take them to Israel.

When it was nearly time to go, the sheik and his wife asked to speak to me privately before I left. They took me to their bedroom, a large chamber containing a tremendous Persian carpet and a handsome four-poster bed. Inwardly I groaned at the prospect of having to accept more of their gratitude. Perhaps the operation had brought about the remission of the sheik's symptoms, or perhaps his faith in the American doctor was what had caused that happy effect. It was not for me to destroy that faith, and so I waited patiently. At last the wife began, shyly, to speak.

"My husband and I have been married for nine years," she said, "and although we love each other very much and are very fond of children, Allah has not blessed us with a child. Is there anything that you know of that we might do?"

At the hospital before his operation the sheik had described his symptoms as having "contaminated" his life. Now I knew what this proud man had been alluding to. How much effort he must have had to make to admit to this difficulty so that we might discuss it. The problems of fertility were not my specialty, but no one could have turned away from the sincerity and concern of this couple. We talked about their situation for fifteen or twenty minutes. Nothing seemed to be fundamentally wrong. Perhaps anxiety and illness were the only barriers to conception, I thought, and proceeded to encourage them to look hopefully on the situation.

(The American doctor's advice, or human nature—probably the latter—turned the trick. About a year later I received a triumphant cable from the sheik announcing that his wife was pregnant. When Helen and I came to Israel two years afterward, the couple came to Tel Aviv to show the American doctor and his wife their baby.

"My husband insists it was the operation that made it possible," his wife said. "He felt so vigorous, you know."

"He may be right, although I've never heard of that happening," I replied. I couldn't help but smile. "Anyway, you have a fine baby, and that's the most important thing."

You could see that she agreed wholeheartedly.)

After the consultation in the bedroom that night, we were served a delicious, very sweet cake with coffee and oranges from a grove belonging to the sheik. About nine o'clock we said good-bye. My Israeli companions looked like contented children. Not for many months had they had so satisfying a meal. Nazareth was autonomous and not restricted to rationing like the rest of Israel.

On the way back to Tel Aviv, a plane flew overhead. It reminded me of "the magic carpet" once more, and I mentioned my desire to go on one flight.

"But the planes are crewed by *goyim*," one of the Ministry of Health doctors said. "It would be dangerous for a Jew to take the trip."

"Never mind all that," I said stubbornly. "I want to go anyway. I want to go on one of those flights."

He was silent, but I had a feeling that he would try to press my case with the authorities. Sure enough, a few days before I was due to leave, Yan Yanai came to the hotel.

"They've decided to look the other way and let you go on one of these missions," he said.

He shook his head in disapproval. "It's strictly unofficial. The risk and responsibility are all yours."

"Thanks, Yan," I said. "I understand about the responsibility being mine, of course."

"All right," he said. "Go buy yourself a uniform like the ones the pilots you see in the bar here wear. Put it on tonight. Sometime after midnight someone will call your room. Be ready for him."

"Tonight!" I said. "I'll be ready. Thanks so much for this. You don't know how much I appreciate it."

"Damn fool thing for a man your age and with your skills to be risking," he said brusquely, but then he added, with a faint smile: "Wish I were going with you."

When the phone rang at about two in the morning I was ready and waiting in an ill-fitting uniform and peaked cap that was too big. An airport limousine stood in front of the hotel. Only the driver and another man were in it. They asked no questions and we drove silently to the airport, where a man who looked like a pilot met me at the entrance.

"You're Dr. Rosen?" he asked.

"Yes."

"Glad to have you with us," he said. "Now, you stick close to me all the time. Wherever I go, you just come along. Don't say anything, don't worry, and let me have your passport."

He hurried me out to where the twin-engine plane stood in the darkness. Inside, boards had been laid across the aisle from one row of bucket seats to the opposite row. This makeshift arrangement changed the seating capacity from about fifty persons to about a hundred.

In the cockpit, the pilot, co-pilot, and crew chief ran through their checks of the plane's mechanical condition. The old engines roared to life promptly and reassuringly, and we taxied out to the runway and took off. Once we were airborne, the co-pilot left his seat and motioned me to take it instead. Soon the sun would rise.

"We're going to Iran," the pilot said, handing me his chart.

It was like going back to high school. The map showed the cradle of Western civilization. Here was a light blue line, labeled "Euphrates R." Further along our course another wavering line bore the legend "Tigris R."

We were flying eastward over Jordan into Iraq, destination Teheran. The sun rose over Iraq directly in our path of flight, flaring red against the windshield. Below, the sands that cover cities thousands of years old crawled slowly beneath the plane. The names of Ur, Nineveh, Babylon flashed into my mind. I remembered with a grin that the Code of Hammurabi established surgeons' fees four thousand years ago. If the surgeon killed his patient, the Code required that his right hand be cut off. It occurred to me that things could be worse.

In the distance, as the sun rose higher, a tiny line of blue meandered through a green valley. I pointed to the Euphrates on the chart and received a confirming nod from the pilot. Beyond lay the Tigris, but the pilot turned the plane southward.

"We're not supposed to fly over Baghdad," he said nonchalantly, "but we don't often have distinguished passengers."

We flew within sight of the city that had once dominated Asia Minor and held sway all across North Africa and the Iberian peninsula. I was looking down at the city where Caliph Harun al-Rashid once ruled, the city of the *Arabian Nights*. We had been flying about three hours now. In two more we were letting down to land at Teheran.

At a little airport, the pilot taxied up to a place where hundreds of men, women, children, and infants were penned in two wire enclosures like cattle. An argument followed with the authorities.

"You can't board any of them," the official said. "We have papers for one hundred and one, but there are one hundred and three in that pen."

The pilot would not be put off with this. He investigated. What had happened was that, during the interminable weeks of processing, two babies had been born. Fearing that the Iranians would not permit the newborns to go along with their parents, the refugees had not reported the births.

When the pilot reported the facts to the airport official, that gentleman merely shrugged his shoulders.

"Chief of police in Teheran is the only one who can clear that up."

We drove into Teheran with me staying close to the pilot as instructed. At police headquarters a young soldier armed with a rifle stopped us at the entrance. Finally our reasons for coming were cleared up, and the pilot went upstairs to confer with the chief. After what seemed hours but was only a few minutes, he returned, and we drove back to the airport with authority to load the plane.

"It's overloaded anyway," the pilot said casually, "so what's a few more pounds of baby fat?"

Slowly the people filed into the airplane, pausing in the doorway to look back and wave timorously at those they were leaving behind in the other enclosure. Only the babies did not wave goodbye, and each time a refugee waved, those who were being left behind clapped and cheered.

Inside it was stifling. There were no toilet facilities. The refugees, tired, hot, and dirty, sat down patiently on the boards, holding on to their board or to each other. As I wormed my way to the cockpit I patted the shoulders nearest me. If these people had ever seen an airplane before, it had only been as one flew far above their heads. They were frightened and anxious, yet they waited calmly for take-off.

The heavily laden Dakota ground down the runway as if it would never become airborne, but the pilot had made no mistake. Slowly it reached flying speed and the moment it took off the pilot ordered the landing gear retracted with a brisk upward movement of his thumb. To a mere physician, the gesture looked comically vulgar, as though the pilot was expressing his contempt for the Teheran airport, the chief of police, and especially that uncooperative airport official.

Then came the long flight back, more than 900 miles. In the cabin the heat was overwhelming. People were vomiting. There was no water. After a time, they became so exhausted that they fell over on one another in a half-dazed sleep. They looked like so many cadavers swaying limply in the motion of the airplane. For hours they half lay that way. Ahead of us the sun set over Egypt and the Mediterranean. We flew on into the night. Below us Iraq slipped by unseen. We crossed the Jordan. Then, in the distance, the lights of Tel Aviv. Our passengers began to stir, and whisper to one another. They peered out the dirt-smudged windows on either side. They began to sing and pray. Suddenly I realized they were singing "Shma Israel." Tears came to my eyes as I tried to join in. The plane circled the field and came in for a hard landing. We were home and Israel's population was greater by 103 precious human lives.

That night I lay in the hotel bed, my head still full of the sights, sounds, and feelings that had filled the long day. I had taken an emotional pounding, but I had experienced something that I would never forget. I had shared the critical moment in the lives of a hundred fellow Jews and had crossed that river of hope, the Jordan, with them.

# Of Deaf Muslims, Christians, Hindus, Jews

Sometimes when I tell that "magic carpet" story, the listener will frown, purse his lips, and shake his head slightly in mute disapproval. Wasn't it awfully risky? What possible benefit could a middle-aged ear surgeon get from it that was worth the chance I had taken?

The risk could easily be exaggerated. Those Dakotas may not have been beautiful, gleaming airliners. In fact, they were rather dusty and weatherbeaten. But they shuttled back and forth between Israel and various countries as monotonously as ferryboats in a busy harbor. In Iran, where there was little risk, no one had paid the least attention to me. If they said something to my friend the pilot, he obviously had satisfied them. The bureaucrats of any nation, I have discovered, like the busy, respectable, established members of any profession, have easily satisfied curiosities.

I have not. Once I had seen a little bit of the big world outside the borders of the United States, my curiosity was whetted for more. I wanted to go everywhere and see everything.

You can't do that, though, if you have any sense of responsibility toward your family, your patients, and your profession, so what I did, of course, was to go home, call in my office staff, and resume my practice.

The trip had done me a lot of good. My mental outlook was very different from what it had been when we left. The covert attacks on me at the hospital and the snubs at medical meetings seemed so much more petty when one knew that in another part of the world people were hard at work building a new nation.

As soon as I returned, I got in touch with Moe Bergman and told him about a problem the Israeli otologists had. As a fenestration surgeon, I had asked the Israelis about the incidence of otosclerosis there. No one could answer my questions. No survey had been made of the number of deaf persons or the causes of their deafness, because in the whole country there was no facility where a hearing loss could be scientifically evaluated. Dr. Bergman was the ideal man to lend a hand in such a situation, I told my Israeli colleagues. They asked me to extend their invitation to him when I returned to New York.

Dr. Bergman jumped at the chance. He went to Israel and made a thorough study of the situation there. Then it was his turn to call me up when he got back.

"Sam," he said, "they need a real audiology center, one that has all the modern equipment for diagnosing hearing loss."

He went on to explain that he had elected himself and me as a committee of two to accomplish this somehow, and in time we did. It is still one of the best centers in the Middle East.

Meanwhile, I had settled back into the routine of my rather reduced practice of otology, and particularly of ear surgery. Life went on, thanks to some loyal patients and to other doctors who felt that, regardless of Helen's and my political activities, I was the surgeon they wanted for their patients.

Helen and I often reminisced about the trip. It had been a great idea, I admitted; it had gotten me out of the routine; it had stirred my imagination and given me a perspective about myself and about what was really going on in the world, not just here at home. What a pity we wouldn't be able to do it very often.

Then came Mr. Lawrence with his mobilizable stapes and everything was changed. When I encountered such fierce resistance to the idea at home, it was only natural that I should think of taking my case abroad to England and to Israel. When, finally, the discovery was accepted, invitations from abroad poured into my office. From east, west, north, and south, otologists the world over wanted me to come and demonstrate stapes mobilization. And I had vowed to myself that never would I refuse a legitimate request to come and teach this new method of restoring hearing.

That vow resulted in my traveling not only all over the United States and Canada but to many foreign lands. By this time we had laid down a few ground rules for these trips. My office would be closed about three months a year for this purpose, but my staff continued on full pay. Outside of New York, no fees would be accepted. Since no hospital abroad would be likely to have the twenty-five or so instruments that I needed, we would take a set along for my own use plus extra sets to leave behind at each place. The instruments, most of which I had designed myself, would be gifts to the hospital, but with one condition: any instrument maker in the country was to have the right to study them for the purpose of manufacturing them for use in that country or elsewhere.

Those instruments were heavy. Since we were paying our

own way, it occurred to me that it would be convenient if my tailor could add extra pockets to the lining of my overcoat to hold sets of them. He did a splendid job, and thereafter I walked onto and off airplanes with the special dignity that befitted the "American ear doctor." There was only one slight drawback. Since I am only 5 feet 7½ inches tall and not exactly slender, the overall effect was that in reality I looked rather more like a gray-haired, overcoated teddy bear than a stately surgeon.

There was another, very special ground rule for these expeditions. Helen always came with me. When we first began making these trips abroad, we discovered that many hospitals were reasonably well equipped, but that they had no one who knew how to set up the operating room properly. Helen, who had worked with me on research, proved to be a very quick study. In no time at all, she had mastered the whole preparatory procedure and could, when called upon, act as my operating room nurse as well. This was of great importance not only to me but to the doctors whom I was teaching and the patients on whom I operated. Stapes surgery is delicate. To do it correctly, the surgeon must be completely relaxed, unworried, and unharried by trivial mishaps of the kind that can occur if everything in the operating room is not properly set up for his work. Even then one can become very tense when things fail to go as well as one hopes. When that happens to me, I put down the instrument I am using and deliberately practice the art of muscular relaxation. In my experience, the muscles of the feet are the best indicators of whether all tension has gone out of my body. When my feet are wholly relaxed, I pick up the instrument and go back to work. It's probably just an idiosyncrasy, but I have found that I can best judge the muscular tension if I wear a pair of worn old slippers with wooden Dutch soles, and these are, thanks to Helen, always on hand (or rather, on feet), where I operate.

One invitation to demonstrate stapes mobilization quite naturally came from my friends in Israel. They had not been very enthusiastic about the procedure when I showed it to them earlier, but now they were fully convinced. I accepted. I also accepted an invitation to teach at the Medical College of the University of Cairo, despite the objections of some of my friends.

Before I left for Cairo, a gentleman from the Jordanian Embassy in Washington called on me. Amman had learned, he explained, that I was going to Egypt to teach my new surgery. Would it not be possible to come to Jordan while I was there? He didn't mention that taboo word "Israel."

"No, I'm afraid I don't have time," I said. "You see, I am due in Israel after I leave Egypt, but you know what a nuisance it is to go from Cairo to Jerusalem—Israeli-held Jerusalem, I mean, of course. I have to fly from Cairo to Beirut, wait for hours, then to Cyprus, wait even longer, and then finally to Jerusalem."

"But you will be so close, doctor," the emissary said, "couldn't you possibly . . . ?"

"Well, yes, I could possibly do it. I'll tell you what: It's about sixty feet from the Jordanian sentry post at the Mandelbaum Gate in Jerusalem to the Israeli guard on the other side. Now, I'll be glad to walk those sixty feet, if your government will see that I am driven from Amman to the sentry post. That will give me two days in Jordan to demonstrate my operation."

The Jordanian gentleman left, saying he would ask his superiors. In a day or two he called to say that it had all been arranged. Would I kindly call on the Jordanian consul to have our passports visaed?

I took them around to the consul, but when that worthy opened them and saw the Israeli visas, he handed them back.

"I am sorry, doctor," he said frowning. "Regulations prohibit my visaing these passports. I will have to ask you to be kind enough to obtain new passports without Israeli visas in them."

Could it be that he didn't understand what arrangements had been made? I was dumbfounded.

"You do understand that I am going to Jordan at the specific, formal request of your government and of your leading medical men?" I asked.

"But of course!" he replied, beaming cordially, "and we are most anxious that you come and demonstrate your wonderful surgery for the deaf."

"Well, there is my passport and my wife's. You will either visa them or you won't. I don't care, but your superiors may have other ideas."

He handed the passports back to me, holding them so gingerly that one would have thought they contained deadly germs.

"I shall, of course, take the matter up with my superiors," he said stiffly.

"You do that," I said, and left without further discussion.

Why did you let yourself in for that? I asked myself. I had half a mind to cancel the trip. I hate that kind of stupid nationalism or racism or whatever you want to call it. If I got over there, they would probably make it very clear that I wasn't really welcome. It would be crazy to expose myself and Helen to that kind of thing. But then the importance of teaching stapes surgery crowded into my mind, pushing every other consideration to one side.

The Jordanian consul referred our passport "problems" to the Ambassador in Washington, who perhaps cabled Amman. In any event, within a few days the consul's man called at my office, picked up our untouchable passports in his bare hands, and returned them with Jordanian visas stamped in them despite the presence of Israeli visas elsewhere in the same document. He didn't look too pleased at having to run such an errand.

We were met in Cairo by a young otologist, Dr. Aly el-Mofty, who proved both cooperative and able. Everything had been prepared in advance, so that I was able to begin operating and doing cadaver demonstrations immediately. Toward the end of our stay in Cairo, the U.S. Ambassador invited us to lunch. He was a pleasant career diplomat who congratulated me on the goodwill I was creating for the United States in Cairo.

"I understand you have been invited to meet President Nasser," he said. Of course, he went on, this was a great honor and rather unusual, under the circumstances. He hoped that I would keep in mind the delicateness of the situation here in the Middle East, and especially that I would refrain from bringing up the subject of Israel.

"I'm here as a surgeon," I assured him, "not as a diplomat or a politician."

Nasser's personal physician and Dr. el-Mofty escorted me to the Presidential Palace for the interview. The Egyptian leader was a tall, youngish man who looked as if he would make an ideal end for the Green Bay Packers or the New York Jets. Almost a Greek god, he was broad-shouldered, thick-set in the neck, with a large chest, muscular build, and long legs. He was a diabetic, but his physician had taken such good care of him that none of the effects of the disease were visible then. He looked at me directly with his very dark brown eyes, shook hands, and invited me to sit down at a low table where coffee was ready.

"Thank you for coming here to help my people," he said very directly and simply.

"You are most welcome," I said. "Frankly, I am just a bit surprised that I was invited. I am Jewish, you know."

"Yes, we know that," he said, "but you are here as a

doctor. You are a scientist and a healer. We are not concerned with the fact that you are a Jew, and besides we are all Semites."

He laughed and indicated that we were to be served. We talked for about an hour. Dr. Aly el-Mofty had impressed me greatly, I told him. It was not practicable to teach every aspect of stapes surgery in the short time I had available. Would it be possible for the government to send Dr. el-Mofty to New York for intensive training? Nasser immediately agreed.

"See to it," he said to an aide.

We had changed our air travel plans. From Cairo we flew to Amman, the Jordanian capital, where I spent two busy days operating and teaching. Then, as they had agreed, Jordanian officials put us in a government car and drove us to Jerusalem and the Mandelbaum Gate. Across the no-man's-land between the Jordanian outpost and the Israeli border we could see people waiting to receive us. Our Jordanian escorts unloaded our baggage and carried it over the intervening space while we walked through the gate into the welcoming arms of Teddy Kollek, the Mayor of Israeli Jerusalem, and some of our otological friends of earlier visits.

"The Prime Minister wants to see you," Teddy Kollek said, grinning. We thanked the Jordanians and drove off in the Mayor's car. Ben-Gurion, white-haired and good-humored, received us in his study.

"I understand you saw President Nasser," he said to me at one point.

"Yes."

"Did you talk to him about the Israeli question?"

"No," I said lamely. "I didn't."

He listened as I explained the briefing given me by the American Ambassador.

"And Nasser didn't mention Israel either," Ben-Gurion observed.

"No, he didn't."

The Prime Minister's white mane shook as he laughed heartily:

"Somebody briefed Nasser, too."

Israel was already showing the signs of change. The vigorous pioneering spirit was still there in the countryside, especially in kibbutzim, where men and women loved, worked, and fought side by side, sharing as equals all the hardships, the hazards, and the joys of building their own and their children's lives. But the emphasis had changed. Industrialization of Israeli society was more noticeable. The Israelis born in the British protectorate looked down on immigrants from Europe and America, while they, in turn, considered themselves superior to the Jews who came from the Arab countries. It was all too human and all too familiar to an American. At the bottom of the social totem pole were the Yemenite Jews and other immigrants from Arab lands.

In the operating rooms of the country, however, all these distinctions vanished, as they do everywhere. Attention focused on dealing with the patient's problems, whoever he might be. Working in Israel, I became acutely conscious of the fact that there was really no difference between their medical workers and those of Egypt or Jordan or, for that matter, the Japanese, the Indians, the Russians, or the Americans.

There was the same intense dedication to helping one's fellow man and to studying the nature of disease processes in order to find better ways of coping with them. It didn't make any difference whether the operating room was in New York, Moscow, Cairo, Tokyo, Düsseldorf, Barcelona, Delhi, or Kabul. Jerusalem and Amman, separated by a chasm of hostility, intrigue, and fear, were only forty-odd miles apart. Yet at any moment of the day, men and women in white were bending over the sick and the dying with exactly the same solicitude, the same worried look of strain on their masked faces.

This much we learned as we went from country to country: people are very much the same wherever you go, and they are much better than you expect them to be. By "same" I don't mean that there is anything monotonously uniform about the different nationalities, ethnic groups, and races of this spaceship we call Earth. On the contrary, the variety is utterly amazing, but so is the variation one can see if he walks down any busy street and *really looks* at the passers-by. The human family is very rich in its variety. No question about that. What I am talking about is an identity under the skin. After all that I've seen of our species, I am convinced that this is a fact. Meanness and hostility, hatred and the lust for vengeance—all those things are part of the human make-up beyond a doubt; but so are kindness, gentleness, love, curiosity, and all those traits that we allow ourselves to admire once in a while.

From infancy most of us have been subtly taught that all the good qualities belong to our group. Only other people are evil. It turns out, though, when you meet them that they are just as human as we are, just as good and just as evil. Once again, the question is, What is the fact and what the opinion? The family of man is the fact. Nationalism, racism—those are manifestations of opinions. Sooner or later, if the species survives, the fact is going to prevail; the fact is going to dictate the way in which our posterity will really inherit the earth.

In some parts of the world people know this already. America is cordially disliked in many places, but we ourselves rarely experienced this dislike personally. People always made the distinction between our government, which they feared and mistrusted, and individual Americans. We felt more at home in Delhi, for instance, than in Montgomery, Alabama, where we joined the march from Selma during the civil rights demonstrations of the 1960's, because in Montgomery we could sense the hatred directed at us personally, whereas in Delhi and Bombay we knew that life was as deep and bitter a struggle for almost every man as it was for the blacks of the American South. Even the police of India we preferred to Alabama's upholders of law and order so-called. In Bombay I operated on the chief of the secret service, a giant of an olive-skinned man. When we left, he came to the airport to see us off. I asked him how he was.

"I can hear the birds sing," he said, smiling. A policeman —and something of a poet.

# Of Sound and Silence

When we first began traveling all over the world to demonstrate the new ear surgery, I had hoped that we would get financial support from a foundation. Neither Helen nor I has ever been much good at asking for money, not even when it was for someone else or for some cause we considered worthwhile. We had each been taught to share, not to take. On Grape Street in Syracuse, no one who came to our door was ever turned away empty-handed, no matter how poor we might be. My mother always went to the cupboard, reached into the teapot where she kept money, and handed the visitor something. It was always that way in our house, and I'll bet you the money my mother gave away was the equivalent for the Rockefellers of a billion dollars. That was money we *needed*. Now. For food. What do the Rockefellers need money for? I'll tell you. For power. They say that the very rich never carry any money on them, and I believe it. Money has a different meaning for them. It's not for buying things you need or that your baby needs. It's for something else. You have the cook or the housekeeper order the groceries, and the store charges it, and you pay whenever you happen to get around to it, because you know those tradespeople won't dare risk offending you by asking for prompt payment.

When the rich give money, they do it in style. They give to very worthy causes: museums, hospitals, universities. There is nothing wrong with that. I have known some very fine people who have given most generously to help the sick, to advance medicine, and other such things.

It's very different from teapot or sugarbowl giving, just the same, and the difference lies in what is being given. When Grape Street people gave a quarter or a dollar to somebody on the block who had had bad luck, it wasn't only a gift of the money. It was a gift of ourselves. We would have to scrimp because of it, and the recipient knew that. But more important, the very act said, We know how it is to fall on hard times; we know it's not your fault that things have turned out badly; we know it could happen to any of us. It said, Don't worry, we'll stand by you, we'll stick with you.

After I had made a few ineffectual efforts to get philanthropic money for my teaching trips, I dropped it. I would go ahead on my own. When I came back from my first trip teaching stapes surgery, I had spent quite a bit in hard cash and had lost more than that, if you count the two to three months when I could have been operating steadily on the patients who flocked to my door, once the discovery of stapes mobilization had been recounted in the magazines and newspapers.

This was something Helen and I wanted to do, and we really wanted to do it ourselves, just for the sheer pleasure of doing it, for the adventure of it, and for the satisfaction of giving ourselves to other people all over the globe. We stopped asking anyone for help, but I couldn't resist telling wealthy patients about the work we were doing. Most of them would listen politely, even attentively, and then make some innocuous comment. It was interesting. About one out of ten would offer to contribute, and that always thrilled me. Here was a person who was not going off to some far land with us. He was not going to share our experiences, except very indirectly. Yet he had the imagination and the compassion to see those people, thousands of miles away with the mute plea for hope in their eyes, and the doctors in those countries so anxious to learn how to help their people in this way. When someone pulled out his checkbook without even being asked, without even a hint, I felt almost as if I were a patient whom he had restored to health. I feel close to those wonderful people, because their gifts mean they understand me, they know why I do what I do. They have given me that understanding.

Of all the people who have given me the gift of self, Helen comes first. This is not a personal memoir, strictly speaking, and I have therefore refrained from going into the more intimate aspects of my life. Don't worry; I'm not going to start now.

Helen and I have shared everything: the good, the bad, times of real fear, times of warmth and joy. Nothing ever got Helen down, even things that have had me so discouraged and depressed that she had to drag me out of them by doing things like renting the house and booking passage to Europe. Helen is game for everything. When I got back from one trip to Europe, the first thing I said after we embraced was, "How would you like to go to the African jungle?"

"When do we start?" she said. It wasn't really a question, and she meant it absolutely seriously. Good thing, too, because I really had decided we would have to mount an expedition to a remote part of Sudan.

During our travels and at home we had seen a great deal of conductive deafness, due to otosclerosis or other causes such as hereditary defects or damage to the middle ear. We had also often come upon cases of nerve damage, children born with defective hearing, war veterans and others who had sustained injury to the inner ear by fracture of the temporal bone, victims of the ignorant or stupid administration of toxic drugs that destroyed or damaged the cochlear nerve. There was nothing we could do for these people, but more and more we became interested in nerve deafness. What was it? Oh, sure, it was, by definition, deafness that showed up in bone-conduction audiograms, deafness that was due to some impairment of the inner-ear mechanism, presumably the organ of Corti with its delicate basilar membrane and its complex—fantastically complex—winding staircase of hair cells and their associated neurons leading inward and upward into the cerebral cortex of the brain.

Nerve deafness does not come only by heredity or injury, however. It comes to everyone who lives long enough. As the decades of life pass, hearing acuity declines. For some the slope is steeper than for others.

Why? Why should it be like that? The obvious answer was that the organ of Corti wears out like other body parts. But scientists take nothing for granted. The right question was, *Does* it wear out? And if so, Why did one person's hearing decline faster than another's? We thought about this carefully, debating it on planes and trains, in hotel rooms. We read the literature to see what answers others might have to the same question.

Well, let's see. If something wears out in the inner ear, what would cause the wear? Why, noise, of course. Studies had shown that at factories, construction projects, jet airports, and on other noisy jobs, workers suffer irreversible neurosensory hearing loss. Protective ear muffs and plugs only prolong the process by slowing it down.

But what about the constant noise of everyday life in our highly mechanized society? What happens to the dweller in

Megalopolis exposed to the roar of traffic, aircraft, sirens, motorcycles, trucks, jackhammers, riveters, subways—and rock music at maximum volume?

We didn't know what happens, because when we first started working on this question, there was no way to compare a population living in, say, New York or Moscow, with one living in a really quiet environment. *Really* quiet, I mean. One in which the average ambient noise was hardly above the decibel level of a whisper, an almost silent world.

We did have some clues, however. Men's hearing acuity declines more rapidly than women's in industrial societies, since men tend to work at jobs involving greater exposure to noise. The trouble with this kind of observation is that it is very inexact. One has no chance to see whether, in actual fact, the men whose hearing is studied really do work in noisier environments.

What to do? Helen and I pondered the problem and talked with otologists and researchers in the physiology of hearing in many countries. There was no apparent solution.

Then one day I was in Düsseldorf as the guest of Dr. Dietrich Plester (nicknamed Peter). After dinner we were chatting in his study when I noticed that he had a gun. The conversation turned to hunting.

"I shot a lion once," he said. "We were on an expedition in Ethiopia where I was doing some ethnological studies. We had a Jeep and came upon a lioness with her cubs. She rushed the Jeep and I fired. I killed her, but unfortunately for me, she clawed my arm and shoulder very badly. We drove straight on to where our guide said there was a mission hospital in the jungle. It was about fifteen miles across the border in Sudan. The region is occupied by a stone age culture called the Mabaan. Marvelous people, Sam, absolutely marvelous."

Some instinct prompted me to ask him to tell me more.

"Oh, they are tall, mostly naked, erect, sinewy, very

peaceful and friendly. Their remoteness from everything civilized seems to have made them in many ways more genuinely civilized than the men we think of as 'civilized.' "

Erect, friendly, civilized. I shut my eyes, picturing the jungle scene. I had been thinking about the noise research problem, so I asked: "Is it a quiet place?"

"Utterly," said Dr. Plester. "They don't beat drums. They don't war on other tribes. They have one five-stringed musical instrument. I would guess the loudest sound they ever hear is thunder and occasionally the roar of a beast."

"Peter!" I exclaimed, "that's what we've been looking for for years: a population like this where there's an almost noiseless environment."

My colleague caught my enthusiasm. We began planning the expedition right then and there. To get to the Mabaan country, we would have to travel overland by Jeep in the dry season. Peter knew of a Jeep for sale in Khartoum. I gave him my check to buy it.

Back in New York, I called on the Sudanese Ambassador to the United Nations, told him about my teaching of stapes surgery, and offered to teach it in Khartoum, provided I and my party would be allowed to go to the Mabaan country to study the tribe. He would try to help, he said, but who and where were the Mabaans?

We found out the answers to those questions the hard way. The Mabaan country is some 600 kilometers almost due south of Khartoum. Eventually, not one but three expeditions resulted, because each time we worked our way back to what a science writer in *Life* magazine—Albert Rosenfeld—called "Dr. Rosen's Shangri-La," we found more things to study.

There were lots of problems. Getting permission proved to be the easiest part. Then came the business of organizing the logistics of a scientific expedition involving transporting ten men and a woman to a jungle region far from any source of power, without refrigeration, without any of the means we were so accustomed to use in running audiometric tests, processing and preserving samples of blood, and taking electrocardiograms—not to mention the stark but remarkably complex problem of assuring an adequate food supply. But Helen was up to the task. Thanks to her ingenuity and the know-how and unreserved cooperation of the Sudanese Ministry of Health, all went well.

When we reached the tribal village of Boing on our first trip, it proved to be, if not a novelist's idea of Shangri-La, then an otologist's dream of one. We measured the background noise in the center of the village with a Rudmose noise analyzer. The sound level was about one-tenth of that emitted by an electric refrigerator.

Even before we began testing their hearing, it was obvious that the Mabaans heard well. They walked along the trails single file, sometimes separated by as much as 100 yards, the length of a football field. Yet they conversed in normal tones. The one in front did not even turn around to reply!

Once our hosts had gotten to know us, we settled down to the serious business of taking exact measurements of hearing acuity, the amount of cholesterol in blood serum, blood pressure. Everywhere we measured the environmental noise level, except in one case. On the second trip, Dr. Aly el-Mofty, the Egyptian otologist who participated in these studies, noticed that in our camp there was a new element added to the noise level. Dr. Mohamed Halim's notes tell the story:

> The night was pleasant. The weather was cool and no sooner we went to bed than the orchestra of snores was conducted by Abdel Razzak, Dr. Aly el-Mofty, the low, rhythmic tone of Peter intermingled, sometimes damped down by Sam's high-pitched, continuous snore, all in harmony with Satti's reaching from a distance. Aly el-Mofty tried to set up the Nagra [tape recorder] for recording, but Sam did not approve of it.

We had decided that the minimum number of Mabaans we must test in each ten-year age group (or decade) would have to be 100. Only in that way could we have a statistically sound set of data which we could then compare with subjects in the same age group tested in widely scattered parts of the world—Düsseldorf, New York, Cairo—and with the results of earlier testing done, for example, at the Wisconsin State Fair by Dr. Aram Glorig.

It will come as no surprise when I report that the Mabaans aged fifty to fifty-nine had better hearing than Americans aged twenty to twenty-nine. Much more significant, however, was the fact that the Mabaans' ability to hear high frequencies, 14,000 cycles per second, for instance (a higher note than the topmost piano key), declined very slowly with age. As age increases, fewer and fewer members of an urban population can hear a tone of this frequency. When the pitch is stepped up to 16,000 and 18,000 cycles, the decline is even more striking. But in the Mabaan tribe, a few men and women over seventy could hear the thin, high-pitched sound.

These were exciting findings, but what did they mean? On the three expeditions, we brought with us various specialists to study other factors. Drs. el-Mofty, Plester, and myself were otologists. To round out our investigation, we asked a Sudanese epidemiologist, a cardiologist, an internist, an ophthalmologist, and a psychiatrist to accompany us. With their aid we confirmed what we had suspected almost from the outset. We had noticed that the Mabaan man of seventy-five had the same blood pressure as the Mabaan of fifteen, about 115/65. By contrast, the mean blood pressure of healthy American men rises, on the average, from about 120/65 to 160/80. The blood pressure differences between Mabaan women and American women are almost as striking. The African tribe was also completely free of the diseases we associate with ageing in Western civilization. Their teeth showed almost no signs of decay. Once when we mislaid the bottle-opener, a Mabaan clenched the cap between his strong, regular teeth and removed it. Most striking was the complete absence in the tribe of vascular hypertension (high blood pressure), coronary thrombosis (heart attacks), duodenal ulcer, ulcerative colitis, acute appendicitis, and bronchial asthma. Electrocardiograms indicated that there was none of the reduced blood supply to the heart muscle, even in elderly Mabaans, that often accompanies the ageing process in Europe and America. We also found that their blood serum had very low cholesterol levels.

This was not a surprising finding. The Mabaan diet is not very exciting, and certainly not what you would call rich. The staff of life in Mabaan country is a sour, fermented bread made of millet seed and water. Occasionally they would vary this with very meager catches of wild fowl, small animals, nuts, and so on. At harvest time they drink large amounts of a beer made from the millet seed.

It may not sound appetizing, and a nutritionist might shake a professional head at such a diet. Yet we found no signs of malnutrition: no rickets, no beri-beri. Instead, we found indications that the diet and perhaps heredity had given the oldest Mabaans very young arteries; so young, in fact, that Dr. Mohamed Hamad Satti, one of our Sudanese colleagues, contended from the beginning that our estimates of the age of our subjects—based on eruption of teeth, signs of puberty, and other data—were too low. He thought that we were understating their ages by several years. If he is right, this would make all the more remarkable the differences between the blood pressures and hearing acuity of Mabaans of each age decade when compared to the same measurements in men and women of the same age groups living in the megalopolises of Western civilization.

To cover a further factor as well as noise levels, diet, blood cholesterol, electrocardiograph readings, and health histories, we added still another specialist on our third trip. He was a Sudanese psychiatrist, Dr. A. T. Bashaar. We wanted him to tell us whether there were severe, moderate, or no signs of psychological stress among the Mabaans. Was life, from their point of view, hectic, anxiety-producing, full of danger and fear? How many of them had signs of mental disease? Dr. Bashaar interviewed our subjects by the hundreds. He could find only one woman who he thought might be psychotic. As for general psychological stress, his skillful interviews showed that the Mabaans were marvelously free of mental strain and stress. They never went to war. On the rare occasions when men fought each other, it was almost always over a woman. The lives of the Mabaans moved in an even tenor.

We came to think of these remote tribesmen as possessing a very deep biological wisdom, a profound knowledge of how to live with nature that members of more complex societies have lost. The Mabaans' biological clocks kept smoother and slower time than Western man's. Their lives harmonized with the rhythms of sunrise, sunset, the change of seasons, the slow, almost undetected passage of the years. They still possessed the wisdom of an ancient Chinese, Lao-tzu, who in the sixth century before Christ wrote in *The Way of Life*:

*Those who flow as life flows know*
*They need no other force:*
*They feel no wear, they feel no tear*
*They need no mending, no repair.*

# Of Hearing and the Heart

--------------------------------------------------------------------------------

Our Mabaan reports inspired a single, fascinating case report in a medical journal by Dr. A. J. Philipszoon of Amsterdam, Holland. He had examined an eighty-two-year-old man before prescribing a hearing aid. In the left ear canal, the doctor found a large brownish mass so impacted in the canal that it could not be flushed out and had to be removed with a forceps. It was a thirty-two-year-old piece of cotton that some doctor had forgotten to remove when the patient had had an earache.

What an opportunity! The man was a walking laboratory for the study of presbycusis, the loss of hearing acuity in the nerve as a function of age. One ear had not been exposed to noise for thirty-two years; the other had. Seizing the chance, Dr. Philipszoon found that a bone-conduction audiogram of the left, unobstructed ear showed pure perceptive (nerve) hearing loss. In the right ear, bone-conduction tests revealed markedly higher acuity.

Each time the members of the expedition to the Mabaan country returned to Khartoum, Cairo, Düsseldorf, New York, we compiled our data, set it up in comparative tables, converted the results to graphs showing the curve of hearing loss with age, and began the laborious but essential process of statistical analysis. The last item sounds dull, but it is not. Differences in data do not necessarily mean anything, because some differences can merely be the product of chance. Statisticians have ways to calculate whether a particular difference is greater than pure chance and if so to what extent.

In medical science, we are usually forced to study things as we find them. We can't arrange a nice, neat experiment and carry it out repeatedly under exactly controlled conditions. The very existence of the Mabaans, for example, is such an experimental situation, but unfortunately it was not possible to compare only the effect of silence in their surroundings with the effect of the roaring traffic's boom on the creatures who walk the sidewalks of Khartoum, Cairo, Düsseldorf, New York. The other factors vary also. The chief of the Mabaans differs rather markedly in countless ways from Mayor Lindsay. So do the Mabaans from the Manhattanites. There are no Mabaans in gray flannel suits, no New Yorkers toting spears down Broadway. No Mabaans gorging themselves in expense-account restaurants, no New Yorkers subsisting quietly on a sour fermented millet paste with an occasional Central Park squirrel thrown in for a special treat. And of course there was no way to set up an experiment involving 1,000 Mabaans and 1,000 Manhattanites so that we could, after a suitable interval of perhaps twenty-five years, check on the results.

Fortunately, a small army of cardiologists, physiologists, and nutritionists had already explored much research territory for us. By studying their preliminary reports of epidemiological research in many parts of the world, we could make some highly educated guesses about the significance of some of the data we had gathered among the Mabaans. For the previous ten or fifteen years, researchers had been looking into the incidence of coronary artery disease in various populations and comparing it with other factors such as psychological stress, the amount of saturated animal fat in the diet, the blood cholesterol level. Gradually, evidence was accumulating that a population whose diet is high in saturated fats has significantly higher blood cholesterol levels, higher incidence of atherosclerosis (hardening of the arteries), higher blood pressures, and higher incidence of coronary artery disease as evidenced by abnormal electrocardiographic tracings or heart attacks or both. By contrast, populations whose diet is low in saturated fats and higher in polyunsaturated vegetable fats seemed to have significantly lower cholesterol levels, blood pressures, atherosclerosis, and coronary disease, when the two populations were compared with due attention to matching age and sex.

By the time our third safari to Sudan was ended, these studies of heart disease and the factors related to it had been quite thoroughly documented in many more studies all over the globe. Furthermore, the experts in that field had reached a consensus that some of these factors indeed did lead to others; that the low-fat diet was related to low cholesterol levels, which in turn were related to low blood pressure, low incidence of atherosclerosis, and consequently to low incidence of coronary disease.

Reading the vast amount of medical literature on these studies convinced me that whatever kind of diet causes high cholesterol levels—and a high-animal-fat diet is certainly one —is closely linked to the premature onset of atherosclerosis. This simplified our problem considerably. Since these studies were carefully reported, we could test the same groups that the cardiologists had, measuring the noise levels in their environments and testing their hearing acuity by ten-year age groups. The results, we reasoned, ought to give us more than a few clues to our new experimental question: Could this cluster of factors—diet, blood pressure, atherosclerosis, coronary disease—have any relation to hearing loss?

One epidemiologic study had been conducted by the University of Minnesota physiologist Dr. Ancel Keys on the Greek island of Crete. The Cretans, except for a higher environmental noise level, had similar factors as the Mabaans in terms of diet, cholesterol, blood pressures, and cardiovascular status. Dr. Keys and his co-workers supplied detailed data of their study, so that Mr. John Guerriero, my staff audiologist, could go to Crete and make parallel hearing studies. When he returned and assembled his data, we were not surprised to see that the Cretans had significantly more acute hearing, age for age, than New Yorkers and other urban populations in affluent communities, but not as acute as the Mabaans.

Still we did not know enough about the diets of our controls from the big cities. We looked around—all around. It seemed Finland was the place to go. The Finns are inordinately fond of milk. Every time you turn round, you are offered a glass, with butter, cheese, bread. In one remote area of eastern Finland, Dr. Keys told me, the population aged forty to fifty-nine is notoriously high in cholesterol levels and atherosclerosis and has one of the highest rates of coronary heart disease in the world. Dr. Keys suggested that we compare hearing acuity there with a matched group of subjects living in the mountains of the Dalmatian coast of Yugoslavia where the opposite conditions obtained. Working with Finnish and Yugoslav researchers, he had investigated both populations and had precise data that would be available to me.

Using our high-frequency audiometer, we studied subjects aged fourteen to twenty-nine in both areas. What we found only whetted our appetite for more research along these lines. The Finns definitely did not hear as well as the Yugoslavs, even though environmental noise levels were about the same.

We longed, however, for a neater experimental setting. And it turned out not to be such an impossible dream after all. While I was in Finland, I had heard about another study that suited the case almost perfectly. A Finnish research group headed by Dr. O. Turpeinen was conducting it in two mental hospitals. In one, the Kellokoski Hospital, they had arranged matters so that the customary milk-and-butter-rich Finnish diet would continue to be the daily fare for a guaranteed five-year period. In the other, Nikkila Hospital, they got a similar guarantee that polyunsaturated vegetable fats would replace most of the animal fat in the diet.

For five years they kept careful track of the patients at both hospitals. The blood cholesterol levels of patients at the Nikkila Hospital fell as soon as the diet was changed and remained significantly lower than those of the patients at Kellokoski. Electrocardiograms of the Nikkila patients indicating diseased coronary arteries were markedly lower. Even deaths from heart attack also fell below those in the other institution, although not enough to be considered statistically significant by Dr. Turpeinen and his associates.

As the five-year period ended, Helen and I packed ourselves and our gear off to Helsinki to study the two hospital populations. Since these were mental patients, we were a little worried about the reliability of their responses to the pure notes they would hear in the earphones of the audiometer. We needn't have been. They understood us perfectly, and cooperated marvelously, even though some of the ways they used to show that they heard the note were a trifle unconventional. Instead of raising her hand, for instance, one dignified patient, who had been a famous prima donna, simply sang the note in her now tremulous soprano.

What we learned had us singing too. Both ten-year age

groups (40–49; 50–59) at the Nikkila (low-fat) hospital had markedly better hearing at all the test frequencies. Differences in hearing acuity in these carefully controlled populations, where we *knew* what the diet was and what the cardiovascular data were, definitely paralleled the differences in diet and coronary disease.

But Dr. Turpeinen and his associates were not finished with their experimental study. They adopted the technique of cross-control; they switched the diets. Nikkila went back on the old high-saturated-fat diet; Kellokoski patients began eating the same diet that the Nikkila patients had been consuming for the past five years.

We waited patiently—well, fairly patiently. At the end of almost four years, we ran a new study. Not all of the patients we had tested at the end of the first five years were still in the hospitals. Some had died; some had been discharged; but since many mental illnesses are unfortunately of long duration, we found a large enough number to give us statistically valid results.

What we learned this time was utterly fascinating. In Kellokoski, blood cholesterol levels had declined; in Nikkila, they had risen. In Kellokoski, the number of *new* cases of coronary artery disease had fallen; in Nikkila, they had climbed. This was perhaps to be expected, but what really amazed us was that in both age groups hearing acuity had definitely improved at Kellokoski while it undoubtedly worsened at Nikkila.

Dr. Turpeinen and his group had concluded by this time that changing the diet of a group is an important factor in preventing coronary heart disease. It was not difficult for Dr. P. Olin, a Finnish otologist who worked with us, and for Helen and me to decide that the same change in diet had reversed the process of hearing loss with ageing.

We were now on a hunt for even bigger game. After comparing the ten- to twenty-nine-year-old eastern Finns with the

Yugoslav youths, and discovering that hearing losses show up at those ages, it had occurred to us that perhaps early hearing loss, or what we might term premature presbycusis, perhaps could be a warning of the onset of atherosclerosis. If so, it would be a sign that could be detected years before the arterial disease began to take its toll in the form of high blood pressure, aged arteries, coronary heart disease, and death from these causes.

We had managed to keep the noise level factor reasonably stable in all these studies, and had found that hearing acuity seemed to go with a good, healthy cardiovascular system untouched by atherosclerosis. Not only that, but it looked as if a drop in hearing might prove to be the earliest sign of the beginnings of circulatory trouble.

Looking back at the results of our Mabaan studies, however, it was obvious that two other variables had to be examined in still other experimental situations. One was mental stress. The Mabaans were as free of this as they were of all the other factors that we now knew were related to presbycusis. The other was high blood pressure.

It seemed reasonable to assume that the mental stress factors at Nikkila and Kellokoski were similar. On the other side of the globe in San Francisco two cardiologists, Drs. Meyer Friedman and Ray Rosenman, had been studying a population of men aged forty to fifty-nine. One group had been selected for their "coronary-proneness" by personality traits. They were the familiar high-powered salesman or executive type: aggressive, competitive, full of drive—or rather, overdrive!—and imbued with a terrible sense of urgency. They lived the well-known American big city "rat race," and, as studies have shown, they paid for it with a higher incidence of coronary heart disease. The other group was chosen for the opposite traits: placidity, willingness to live and let live, reasonable ambitiousness, and a point of view expressed in the New Testament saying: "Sufficient unto the day is the evil thereof."

With the cooperation of Drs. Friedman and Rosenman, Helen studied the hearing of both groups, dividing them into the usual forty to forty-nine and fifty to fifty-nine age categories. There were a lot of problems with the study, but Helen's data suggest that the hearing of the non-coronary-prone, relatively relaxed men was more acute than that of the coronary-prone runners of the rat race; furthermore, as they aged, the gap between them in hearing acuity distinctly widened.

There remained the blood pressure variable. Was it, too, a factor in coronary disease and hearing loss? It would not do to study a population with high blood pressure whose diet was high in fats or whose cholesterol levels were high, because that would confuse the issue. That diet seems automatically to go with rising blood pressures as its devotees age.

When we looked for a place where blood pressures averaged higher and higher with age but where the other factors were low, our hearts sank. Helen and I have become positively addicted to travel, but the likeliest place turned out to be Hokkaido, the northernmost of the Japanese islands. The people in remote parts of Hokkaido live on a predominantly fish and rice diet, but they have unusually high blood pressures on the average. When we looked at the logistics of transporting our specialized equipment by air, rail, and sampan, we knew it was not going to be easy, but we began to plan the new venture anyway.

We never went to Hokkaido, however. Instead, a series of events that had begun back in the 1950's culminated, quite by accident, in our finding precisely the kind of experimental population that we needed much closer to home—in the Bahamas.

In the 1950's when I was demonstrating stapes surgery in India, Helen and I were invited to meet the late Prime Minister Jawaharlal Nehru. It was a pleasant, if somewhat formal, occasion, during which we sipped tea and talked about literature, art, and philosophy. Suddenly at one point Mr. Nehru mentioned that his cousin, Ratan K. Nehru, suffered from conductive deafness. He hoped that it could be arranged for me to operate on his cousin.

That would have been simple enough, except for the fact that the cousin happened to be the Indian Ambassador to Peking. With the United States actively supporting the Chiang Kai-shek government on Taiwan, we knew that it was most unlikely that we would be welcome in Peking. Hong Kong was on our route to Japan, however, so we arranged for Ratan K. Nehru to come there and be operated on in the excellent British hospital.

Immediately after a very good hearing improvement on the operating table, the Ambassador's hearing fell away again. It worried me, but I reassured him. It was only the traumatic effects of the surgery, I explained.

"In ten days or two weeks," I assured him, "after your ear has completely healed, hearing will return."

The Ambassador must have sensed that I could use a little reassurance myself. Soon after I returned to New York, a triumphant cable arrived, announcing that Mr. Nehru's hearing had come back up and was now excellent. That delighted me, but I gave it no further thought. Not so Mr. Nehru. He evidently sang my praises in Peking. Almost before we knew it, we were being asked by the Chinese Medical Society to come to Peking to demonstrate stapes surgery.

The invitation was official and formal. Even if I had wanted to refuse, I would not have done so, because Helen and I had long since decided that, regardless of the problems, we would go anywhere that any qualified person asked us to teach the new techniques. Besides, the prospect of going to Peking, the capital of the world's oldest surviving civilization, was very attractive. What we dreaded was the necessity of going to Washington first. But go we did, and after interminable discussions with narrow-eyed, tight-lipped State Department officials, at last our passports were validated for mainland China.

Excitedly we packed our bags and booked passage for Paris, where Peking's Ambassador to France would visa our passports. Meanwhile, however, a State Department spokesman decided to announce our trip to the press. We were being allowed to go, he explained self-righteously, because the United States was willing to see that American scientific knowledge (of a non-military nature, of course) was made available to others. He managed to imply that the United States was a kindly, benevolent, enlightened land in contrast to the wicked and ignorant Chinese. Perhaps he didn't know that Chinese civilization flourished four thousand years ago when white men in Europe were living in caves and the Americas were undreamed of by them.

The State Department's tactless essay at capitalizing on our trip was soon noticed in Paris and Peking. A lengthy, polite cable arrived from Peking. The Chinese Medical Society regretted to have to advise me that the time was not considered quite ripe for my proposed trip.

Helen and I looked at each other. We were already weary from haggling with U.S. officials, from the excitement of the prospect of going to China, from the packing, and now from disappointment.

"Come on, Sam," Helen said. She selected two of our numerous valises, gave me one and headed for the elevator with the other.

"If not China, then somewhere. Let's get out of here and away from the television and newspaper people."

Almost by chance, we chose a flight to the Bahamas. We could rest there. We tried that, but neither of us is very good at just lying around on beaches. Inevitably, after a few days, I began to poke around the hospital in Nassau, talking to otologists about ear surgery and hearing acuity and to cardiologists about diet, cholesterol levels, coronaries, blood pressures . . .

Blood pressures! They were tragically high among the Bahamians, so high that strokes in the thirty- to forty-year age group are not uncommon. Yet the dietary, cholesterol, and coronary disease factors were not present. They were relatively low. Here was our "Hokkaido," just a few hours' flying time from New York. Now we could study a population in which high blood pressure was the only altered variable.

Since then Helen and I have returned to the Bahamas many times, teaching stapes surgery, making fast friendships, and studying the relationship between high blood pressure and hearing loss. Naturally, we studied the islanders in the same age groups as appeared in our other investigations around the world, and took the same auditory and physiological data. It turns out that the Bahamians have very little atherosclerosis and very little coronary artery disease. Their blood cholesterol levels are low, yet they have very high average blood pressure and a tragic incidence of early death by stroke.

When we compared the Bahamian data with the results of our studies elsewhere, it was evident that they heard more acutely than the Finns or any other group where coronary disease and cholesterol levels were high. Of course they did not hear as well as the Mabaans. No one does, so far as we know.

From these comparisons we concluded that, unlike atherosclerosis, hypertension (high blood pressure) *in itself* does not cause diminution in hearing acuity.

"Here's something odd, Sam," Helen said one day, soon after we had returned from our first study trip to the Bahamas.

We had been poring over the data, analyzing it by age groups, and preparing comparisons with other studies of other populations.

I looked at her notes. It certainly was odd. Bahamians, we already knew, heard distinctly better than many of our other groups. When you compared each age group with the same one in another population, the hearing of the islanders turned out to be better than that of populations where coronary disease was rampant and not as good as, for example, the hearing of the Yugoslavs and Cretans we had studied.

But there was one age group that did not fit the pattern. Some of the Bahamian children did not hear as well as children in a comparison population that was in other age groups inferior in hearing to the Bahamians. This was something worth looking into further. Was it just an accident of the statistics, or did it represent something that was happening to these Bahamian children—something that had not affected their elders? There was nothing in our data to give us a clue, but Helen proposed a theory.

"The Bahamas have only recently been opened up to big-time tourism," she said. "Suppose these children are the first generation to eat a more typically American diet: milk, ice cream, butter, meat. Could that account for this?"

In theory it would, but since we did not really know what diet the children were consuming, it had to remain a theory.

It was not the first time, though, that we had seen that a poor diet could affect adversely the hearing of children. We had gone to Finnish Lapland once, because we knew that the Laplanders live mostly on reindeer meat, probably the leanest and toughest meat that there is, and because the environment is less noisy than most. Once again we found that low-fat diet, low cholesterol, and low incidence of atherosclerosis went datum by datum with measurably more acute hearing.

Here, too, we encountered a group that did not fit the pattern. They were children who lived in Sevitarui far above the Arctic Circle. Their audiograms showed that for their age they were definitely not as sharp of hearing as their parents. The reason seemed to be diet. Although the parents had lived on the standard, low-fat Lapp diet for years, these children were malnourished. Their food had to be flown in and was lacking in many essential elements of good nutrition, such as fresh fruit and vegetables.

Following these clues provided by the Bahamian and Lapland children—the former malnourished by too "rich" a diet, the latter by too skimpy a one—Helen seized an opportunity offered us to study still another population of children. What intrigued us was that their nutrition had already been intensively studied by Dr. George Christakis of Mount Sinai. This time, therefore, we would not have to make guesses about their diet. And this time we would not have to pack our bags and fly thousands of miles. The children were attending a public school on the Lower East Side of New York City. Instead of a jet, Helen could take the subway.

The children did not do well in school. They were not undernourished; they were *mal*nourished. Some were even fat, but their diet failed to supply them with essential vitamins and minerals and was far out of balance. It was low in protein and high in carbohydrates. Testing them, Helen found that they were almost a perfect match in reduced hearing with the nutritionally deprived Lapland children.

We don't know precisely what any of this means. Obviously, we think that it at least suggests that high-frequency hearing tests can pick up the first signs of nutritional poverty. The high frequencies are those that tend to deteriorate first. Conceivably the time may come, after much, much more research into the high-frequency hearing acuity of children, when it will be possible to say, on the basis of such tests, that a given group of children between ten and nineteen are running a significantly greater risk of developing cardiovascular disease by the time they reach their forties or fifties.

# Of Noise

It is clear that the American doctor and his wife have not been idle. I am writing this chapter at a collective farm in Georgia, U.S.S.R. Helen and I have come in order to study another group engaged in manual labor.

When we first came to the Soviet Union to do research, we did so at the invitation of a Soviet medical team which had been studying cardiovascular disease. We hoped to parallel their studies by measuring the hearing of two different groups. One was comprised of clerical workers and middle-level executives whom the Soviet cardiologists reported as having high rates of coronary disease. The others were workers in heavy industry whose muscular way of life apparently kept their circulatory system in much healthier condition than that of their sedentary fellow citizens.

Sure enough, the coronary-prone bureaucrats' hearing, when plotted on a graph by age and frequency, was losing acuity as they grew older at a much faster rate than others we had tested. Unfortunately, the factory workers had even more hearing loss, because they worked in factories which could only be called cacophonous, they were so noisy. Thus, the study came to naught because a variable that we knew affected hearing loss had unwittingly been added to the control group.

Our Soviet colleagues understood our problem, and so now we are studying another group of control subjects, selected to match the clerical-executive Muscovites whom we studied earlier; only this time they are people who do heavy work but not under such noisy conditions. With this data in hand, we hope to make valid comparisons between the two groups.

As long as a man's mind remains active, there is no end to research. Every time he thinks he has the facts he needs to answer a question, those same facts generate more questions. As we have studied presbycusis all over the world, many friends and patients have been generous in offering help. Colleagues in otology and in other specialties have lent valuable aid and advice.

Many of the laymen who have lent a hand have done so on faith—faith in Helen and Sam Rosen, faith in that modern priesthood called Scientists and that modern religion called Science. The quest for truth, the thirst to slake one's curiosity, the drive to answer that recurring question, Now, why did *that* happen?—all these justify their faith; but I should like to pay a small part of my debt to all these good people and to the reader by venturing just a bit beyond the immediate horizons of our current research.

To come on this journey, you will have to pack a small, theoretical valise containing the fundamentals of what we know about the inner ear and how it functions to transduce sound waves into electromagnetic impulses that travel up the nerve fibers to the brain.

Earlier (in the second chapter), I described the air-conduction apparatus of the outer and middle ear, whose function is to transform the vibrations of airborne sound into short, sharp vibrations which set in motion the perilymph (fluid) that fills the inner ear. Now we must consider what happens in the cochlea, the spiral chamber embedded in hard bone, which lies behind the footplate of the stapes. Dividing that spiral tunnel is an elaborately constructed membrane, bearing delicate hair cells from which groups of neurons radiate and combine like the strands of a rope, to form the nerve of hearing. Otologists and physiologists once thought that simple vibratory motion of this apparatus resulted in its transducing mechanical wave action into the electrical activity of the nerve. Today, thanks to the research of Nobel Prize winner Georg von Békésy, we understand in much more sophisticated detail how the inner ear probably perceives frequency, partly as a consequence of the way its structure influences the mechanical vibrations transmitted to it by the stapes.

Dr. von Békésy has shown that for each frequency of sound entering the cochlea a wave that travels along the membrane is created. The lower region of the cochlea responds to most audible frequencies, but the upper parts of the spiral respond only to low tones. As a result, the lower section of this delicate apparatus is the part that gets the most use and the most "wear." This may explain why, when the ear is assaulted by very loud noise at many frequencies, or when it is exposed to more moderate noise levels over the years of a lifetime, the perception of high frequencies is the first to decline.

A brilliant investigator, Meyer zum Gottesberge, has described this effect as analogous to the wear on a stair carpet. The carpet represents the hair cells and their connected neurons. People climbing the "stairs" represent the vibrations at different frequencies in the inner ear. The low frequencies move over the entire carpet, wearing it evenly, but the high frequencies use only the first flight of "stairs." Consequently, the wear on the carpet decreases from the entrance as one goes toward the top of the spiral. As time passes, the parts of this delicate apparatus activated by the higher frequencies are those that receive the most wear and are therefore the first to show the effects of prolonged exposure to noise.

There are other factors that could affect the efficiency of this extremely tiny, delicate inner-ear organ, named the organ of Corti after the nineteenth-century Italian anatomist who first described it. Our retinal rods and cones, our tactile nerves, our taste buds, our olfactory nerves are all embedded in soft tissue through which course millions of microscopic capillary blood vessels that supply oxygen and nutriments and take away waste products and carbon dioxide. The organ of Corti, however, is surrounded by fluid. The membrane and hair cells are isolated from the circulatory capillary bed because they must be. Otherwise, we would hear nothing but an incredible pulsating racket created by the circulatory system.

No such deafening roar of expanding and contracting capillaries is heard, however, even though normal hearing is incredibly acute. Try plugging the ear canals of both ears at the same time by putting your index fingers firmly into each ear. Listen. You will hear a dull, very low-pitched sound. It is the sound of the blood coursing through the precapillary blood vessels in your fingertips.

Since the organ of Corti cannot be directly supplied by the vascular bed in the way other tissues are, the circulatory functions have to be carried out indirectly, through the fluid that fills the inner ear, bathing the basilar membrane, its hair cells, neurons, and other structures. The perceptor organ is thus one step removed from direct access to the necessities of cellular life. Consequently, the efficiency of blood supply to the cochlea becomes much more critical. Anything that impairs it is likely to affect the efficiency of the inner ear.

This picture of the nature of the inner-ear mechanism gives us some clues as to why hearing loss, and particularly high-frequency loss, is associated with atherosclerosis, and why, indeed, it may be the earliest indication of the beginnings of degeneration of the vascular system. If the organ of Corti is so critically dependent upon an effective circulatory system, and if the high-frequency perceptors in the cochlea are the first to be affected by the impact of sound, then it follows that a truly sensitive, precise measurement of acuity at those frequencies can become a very valuable means of studying cardiovascular disease.

High-frequency audiometry in the future can make partners of otologists and cardiologists, who will collaborate to identify those populations which are developing the earliest, still otherwise undetectable signs of cardiovascular disease.

We already know that the inroads of atherosclerosis seem to be reversible by controlling diet. If we can detect in an individual an abnormally swift decline in his high-frequency acuity, or if we can demonstrate that the hearing of a population is below a given norm for high-frequency perception, then the otologic-cardiologic team will be able to point out the desirability of a change in diet. After all, prudent dietary management is the first resource an internist uses in helping a patient who has just begun to develop overt signs of the diabetes he has inherited. The same principles apply to the postponement of the development of atherosclerosis. If they can be applied in a timely way, many lives will be saved and many others prolonged.

For a time I thought that these speculations were just about the last word on the subject at this time, but there remained one other problem that kept bothering me.

When we went to the Mabaan country on the third expedition, we took along two researchers from Dortmund. They were Drs. Gerd Jansen and J. Schulze of the Max Planck Institute of Physiology. Dr. Jansen and his associates had done research on the stress reaction of human beings when suddenly exposed to loud noise, and we wanted them to compare their data taken from experiments with Dortmund factory workers and other subjects with tests conducted on members of the Mabaan tribe.

They set up their equipment in Boing and shattered the normal silence with exactly the same recorded sounds of factory noises in Dortmund that they had used in their earlier study. This time, the subject was a lanky, handsome Mabaan, to the tip of whose finger a harmless little pressure-sensitive cuff had been attached. Two wires from the cup ran to a device called a plethysmograph, that would record on a moving strip chart the fluctuations in volume of that fingertip. Those volumetric readings accurately traced the expansion or contraction of the precapillary blood vessels in the fingertip.

In Dortmund, using the plethysmograph to measure changes in size of the blood vessels, the German investigators found that a sudden burst of noise caused a constriction of the vessels that persisted for a time even after the noise stopped. Interestingly enough, the same noise that caused vasoconstriction in the Germans caused much more tightening of the blood vessels in the Mabaans, but when the noise stopped, the Africans recovered faster than the Germans. We have no proof that this greater reaction and speedier return to normal is due to the fact that the Mabaans presumably have healthier, more elastic arteries, but that is what we believe explains the difference in response. Some of that greater elasticity is probably due to factors such as diet and heredity, but we think a major component in it is the absence of environmental noise.

Noise is more than just a threat to the delicate mechanism of the inner ear. The vasoconstriction demonstrated by the changes in fingertip volume shows that exposure to noise produces a reaction that affects the whole organism. There are reactions other than vasoconstriction. Noise induces psychic and physiologic shock reactions. The noise-exposed subject winces, turns his head, holds his breath, and closes his eyes for an instant. Then his breathing speeds up, the pupils of his eyes dilate, his skin turns paler. Epinephrine from the adrenal glands floods into his bloodstream.

These are all reactions to stress. Furthermore, they are not within the control of the individual. Dr. Jansen found, for example, that when he exposed Dortmund factory workers over and over again to his taped factory sounds—noise to which they were thoroughly accustomed—they still reacted in the same way. The greater the noise, the greater the reaction, sleeping or waking. Even when the subject is warned in advance that the noise is coming, he cannot control his reaction. It is a reflex. Noise-induced stress affects the sympathetic nervous system and the output of certain hormones, particularly epinephrine.

This all adds up to the fact that while *we* may become accustomed to the constantly growing din of daily life, our nervous system and our heart and blood vessels never do. Studies show that even fairly mild everyday stresses—among them noise —can cause significant increases in the level of epinephrine in the blood. This can in turn set up a reaction in the heart muscle, either because of the constriction in the blood vessels or because of an abrupt change in the chemical balance in the muscle.

Several research teams have studied the effects of noise in animals. In San Francisco, Drs. Friedman and Rosenman exposed rabbits to 102 db of "white noise"—meaning a roaring noise that includes all frequencies from 30 to 20,000 cycles per second—for ten weeks. During the test period, the exposed rabbits showed much higher blood cholesterol levels than control rabbits who ate the same food and lived the same way as the exposed animals, except that they were not exposed to noise. When the San Francisco researchers killed the two groups of rabbits at the end of the ten-week experimental period, they found that the noise-exposed animals had developed a markedly greater degree of atherosclerosis than the control animals. In Vermont, Dr. William Raab exposed wild rats to frightening noises and found that in nearly 70 per cent of them the heart muscle had developed patches of dead tissue.

Conversely, silence is golden, as at least one animal experiment shows. It was inadvertently performed in Israel by Dr. B. Zondek, who had a quiet laboratory located in Jerusalem for some years. He noticed that the number of couplings and pregnancies among his experimental rats was remarkably high. Then he had to move to noisy, bustling Tel Aviv. Immediately, the frequency of intercourse and the number of pregnancies in his rats dropped abruptly.

Mice and men are not the same, but I rather suspect that when it comes to lovemaking, the only sound that has positive erotic effect is the lover's soft murmur.

In still another experiment, Drs. M. Lawrence, G. Gonzalez, and J. E. Hawkins exposed experimental animals to noise and then looked for changes in the blood supply to the cochlea. They observed a significant reduction in blood flow and in the number of red blood cells. This meant that the organ of Corti was relatively starved for both oxygen, which is carried in the hemoglobin of the red cells, and nutriments carried in the serum of the blood. Microscopic examination of the sensory cells showed that they had undergone structural changes that impaired their functioning.

In brief, noise-induced stress causes damage not only to the inner-ear mechanisms but to the blood vessels and the heart muscle as well. This may not seem important to a teen-age rock music fan who listens through earphones with the volume on his hi-fi turned up full blast. The immediate effects of such loud noise are literally deafening: the threshold of nerve response rises; the ears ring after the noise ceases; but after some hours or a day, hearing acuity returns to normal. Repeated doses of loud noise, however, can cause permanent loss, usually in the high frequencies. This is no joke. Parents and young people ought to be aware that loudly played hard rock (or any other music or sound) can do lasting and irreversible damage to the inner ear.

At least it is possible to turn down the hi-fi or, if one is a musician, to wear protective ear plugs if one must play night after night at top volume. Other environmental noise is not so easily controlled, its effects are more subtle, and, as I have pointed out, go far beyond damage to the ear alone. Physicians, hospital administrators, and city officials have long known this, at least intuitively, for most hospitals are protected, though very inadequately, by street signs that command HOSPITAL QUIET and by corridor posters showing a pretty nurse with her finger to her lips and the admonition, "Shhhhhh!"

These feeble efforts to protect patients against noise are based on sound physiological and psychological principles. A healthy person exposed to stress can handle it without serious consequences. But suppose the stressed individual is desperately ill. Suppose he has severe coronary artery disease, for instance, so that his heart muscle is already half-starved for life-giving blood. It is conceivable that the sudden stress created by a loud noise could precipitate an outright heart attack in such a patient.

This is an extreme example. Another noise pollution problem exists which is much less dramatic but potentially far more serious. Would you think that a telephone bell could do harm to the body? Dr. Raab was able to demonstrate that the ubiquitous sound also produces increases in the epinephrine secreted into the blood and causes changes in the electrocardiogram pattern! If "Ma Bell" can do this to us, imagine what damage the noise of jackhammers and jets may be causing.

We should not leave it to imagination. What is needed is a concerted research effort to study the physiological effects of environmental noise, not because noise is the only stress inducer in our lives, but because it is one that we can produce experimentally and measure very exactly and, not incidentally, because most noise is man-made and can therefore be man-unmade if we begin to take it seriously as a dangerous pollutant in our environment.

Modern life is full of stresses, all of which contribute to the accelerated ageing process that industrial man is heir to. The evidence we already have suggests strongly that stress as well as diet is an important factor in the premature development of atherosclerosis and coronary heart disease. Other evidence, as yet somewhat fragmentary, suggests that not all failures of the myocardium (the heart muscle) are the secondary consequence of narrowing or blocking of the coronary arteries. Some damage to the myocardium occurs directly. Most cardiologists don't agree with this idea. The traditional view is that, when the myocardium is damaged or fails completely, the cause is always to be found in narrowing or plugging of the coronary arteries.

Recently, a few scientists in this country and elsewhere (notably in Canada and in Soviet Armenia) have been looking at the effects of stress directly on the heart muscle itself. Their results strongly suggest that the traditional concept of the cause of heart attacks is not tenable.

Of course, many attacks are brought on by narrowing or blocking due to atherosclerosis of the coronary arteries. But apparently a significant number are found at autopsy to have occurred despite the fact that the coronary arteries were perfectly capable of supplying the full amount of needed blood to the muscle.

What then? We have some clues. Stress, including noise, causes a shift in the chemical balance of the heart muscle. Such a change is something like what happens when the engine of a racing car is neglected. If the engine is not too gummed up, the car may only be slowed down. But if the engine is already heavily burdened with carbon deposits, sticking valves, and poor ignition timing, then the changes in the engine (that is, the heart) could stop it entirely.

This is a tremendously challenging problem. Using noise

as the controllable variable, it should be possible to investigate very precisely the effect of different quantifiable amounts of noise-induced stress on the sympathetic nervous system, the endocrine system, the blood vessels, and, most critical, the myocardium. Heart disease and stroke are the leading killers of mankind. Research in stress effects promises to tell us a great deal about the underlying causes of these diseases.

# Of Service to the People

----------------------------------------------------------------------------------

For the time being, at least, I have not been able to go any further with studies of noise and stress, much as I would like to do so. Instead, as has happened so often in my life, the unexpected suddenly changed the direction of my thinking and the direction of our most recent travels as well.

Helen and I had wanted to go to China, not only to teach stapes surgery to Chinese otologists, but to see what was happening in a land where so large a part of the human race had embarked on a bold new social experiment. But we were resigned to the fact that it was probably not to be. The Cold War continued endlessly, if unproductively, and the possibility of a renewed invitation to visit China seemed more and more remote as time passed.

Several years before the State Department put its foot in my mouth, thereby thwarting my one chance to make this journey, I had attended an international meeting of otologists that was being held in Leningrad. A group of Chinese ear specialists were present, and I seized every opportunity I could to talk to them. Like the Russians, they were familiar with the literature of European and American medicine. They knew about the Rosen technique and wanted to try it. Before the meeting ended, I packed a set of my instruments carefully and handed it to one of the Chinese ear surgeons.

"I'd like to come to your country and demonstrate the various techniques," I told him, "but it doesn't seem very likely. So why don't you take these back with you?"

He accepted the gifts graciously and assured me that he hoped that the day might soon come when my pessimistic forecasts would prove to be a "false negative" diagnosis of the international political situation. I knew better, of course, but not wanting to be rude, I let it go, and we continued to discuss the details of stapes mobilization and other methods of surgical treatment of otosclerosis. Returning to New York, I told myself that at least I had had the satisfaction of sending some part of my skills to the Chinese profession in the form of reprints of articles about stapes surgery and the instruments.

I never dreamed of seeing those instruments again, but in 1971 they were shown to me at the Fan Di Hospital in Peking. Our dream, which had faded almost to nothing, had suddenly come true.

It began with a letter from the Ambassador of the People's Republic of China in Ottawa. In polite phrases, Ambassador Huang Hua advised me that the Chinese Medical Association had asked him to extend in the Association's name an invitation to visit China as its guest. If I could come to Ottawa, bringing Helen's and my passports, the letter said, the necessary formalities could be completed without further delay. I called Helen to tell her the exciting news and then called the Embassy in Canada to arrange an appointment for the following day.

In Ottawa, over tea, Ambassador Huang and I discussed my forthcoming visit. We would fly to Hong Kong and then take the train to Canton from Shum Chun at the border. Since we were coming as guests of the medical society, all arrangements for transportation, hotels, interpreters, etc., would be taken care of by our hosts, the Ambassador explained.

He rang for an aide, who presented himself immediately. With a courtesy that I have since learned is endemic in China, the diplomat asked whether, perhaps, the aide could take Dr. and Mrs. Rosen's passports to the appropriate official and have them visaed. One would have thought he was asking a favor of a friend rather than giving an order. When the passports were returned to me, Ambassador Huang rose and bade me goodbye.

"We know how long you have wanted to come to China," he said, "and I am so glad that it is now possible."

In New York, Helen and I at once began our preparations. We were old hands at long voyages to strange places, but this was something quite different. We realized that we knew almost nothing about the conditions we would encounter on the mainland. Chinese operating rooms might be reasonably modern, but we could not be sure. Chinese surgical techniques might prove different. We might be called upon to demonstrate stapes surgery only once or twice in each major city, or there might be, as in India, so many waiting patients that most of our time would be taken performing "demonstration" operations.

Debating what to take with us, we decided finally to pack sets of instruments, my loupes, in case no operating microscopes were available, the headlight, in case operating room lighting proved inadequate, and our audiological equipment. A visit of one month would not be long enough to begin a serious study of hearing acuity, but perhaps we could at least arrange a return at a later time for a more extensive study.

I mention these details only because they demonstrate how

upside down is the American view of things Chinese. During the quarter century in which the United States refused to recognize the People's Republic, Americans have come to think of China as isolated and backward. We have imagined it as a country in turmoil, just beginning to emerge from a state of national paranoia. And we have condescendingly thought recently that perhaps we could bring some of our Western enlightenment to this barbaric, uncivilized land.

It was nothing like that. The first visit we made to a major hospital gave us culture shock. Chinese medicine, like the rest of the country's traditions, is thousands of years old—and as modern as tomorrow. Medicine is practiced on a level equal to, and, as we shall see later, in some cases superior to the quality of European or American medical practice. The Fan Di Hospital in Peking, for example, looks no different to a Western physician than Guy's in London or Mount Sinai in New York.

As for stapes surgery, we had a similar surprise. Chinese otologists had informed themselves fully on the subject and were performing various kinds of mobilization procedures as required. Ironically, in the light of my dreams of bringing a new surgical technique to China, it turned out that the need was not very great because otosclerosis is rare in that country. With characteristic courtesy, however, our hosts arranged for me and Helen to watch a mobilization performed with Chinese-made instruments. The surgeon used an operating microscope devised by him and made by local craftsmen. The operation was as skillfully executed as any I have ever seen.

Our hosts also asked me to lecture on stapes surgery in the big cities. Of course I did so, and to good-sized attentive audiences of doctors, but I wonder whether I told them anything that they had not already learned either from experience or from their close reading of Western medical literature.

The day after we arrived in Canton we were joined by two

other American physicians and their wives. They had also been invited by the Chinese Medical Association. There was Dr. Paul Dudley White, the Boston cardiologist who took care of President Eisenhower during his heart attack in the 1950's, and Ina White. Dr. White has been interested in the social aspects of medicine throughout his long career. With him were Dr. E. Grey Dimond, Provost for the Health Sciences and Distinguished Professor of Medicine at the University of Missouri–Kansas City, and Mary Clark Dimond, the daughter of the late Grenville Clark, an American lawyer and advocate of world federalism. Later we were joined by Dr. and Mrs. Victor Sidel of Albert Einstein College of Medicine in New York. Dr. Sidel is chairman of the College's Department of Community Medicine.

It was a diverse group, both in professional interests and in social backgrounds. For the next weeks we traveled together most of the time, talking freely with Chinese physicians and surgeons, many of whom spoke English fluently. But we all spoke the lingua franca of medicine: the language of the stethoscope, the physical examination of patients, blood and urine test results, the electrocardiogram, the audiogram, and the familiar blood pressure measuring instrument whose tongue-defying name in English is sphygmomanometer.

When our trip was over, we all agreed that our preconceptions about Chinese medicine had been drastically revised. No one had made the least attempt to divert us from talking to whomever we pleased, from seeing anything that interested us, or from going wherever we took a fancy. Far from presenting a fearful or suspicious attitude, everyone, from ordinary citizens in the streets and on the communes we visited to doctors who escorted us and the high officials who received us, made us welcome.

It would be presumptuous to expound a lot of firm conclusions as the result of so short a visit to a country of 800 million population. But there are some things we learned and some experiences we had that are worth recounting. Perhaps the most important is that Western medicine has far more to learn from the Chinese than vice versa, not because Western medicine does not offer the Chinese many valuable techniques and much priceless scientific knowledge. It does, of course, but the Chinese have not isolated themselves from medical progress. Their medical libraries are filled with European and American medical literature, including the latest issues of the leading journals. We are the ones who need to learn, because we have been isolated from them, and because the Chinese, capitalizing on the revolutionary fervor that animates everyone, have embarked simultaneously on two extraordinary socio-medical ventures. There, the practice of medicine is a vast social experiment, unprecedented in medical history. Intimately associated with that experiment is another: the consolidation of the accumulated medical wisdom embodied in the traditional practice of medicine in the Orient with the most modern scientific medicine as it has developed in the West.

Soon after the victory of the Communist revolution in 1949 —an event that the Chinese speak of simply but eloquently as "the liberation"—Mao Tse-tung and the government began to stress a new health policy. The traditional medicine of thousands of years was to be combined with Western-style medicine. Mao contended that in the herbal medicine and acupuncture of the Chinese practitioner was a vein of useful therapeutics that had to be extracted by mining this resource. What was probably just as important for the public health of this enormous country was the fact that in the traditional practitioner the government had ready at hand a professional group who had the confidence of the people and who could help to implement the public health policy of the new government. Not only would the Western-oriented physicians learn at first hand about traditional medicine, but the traditional practitioners would come into

244 · The Autobiography of Dr. Samuel Rosen

contact with such modern tricks of the medical trade as urine analysis, diagnostic X-rays, blood tests, electrocardiography, and all the other means by which we seek to know what is going on in the body of a sick man or woman. Furthermore, the traditional Chinese physician possesses an indispensable ingredient in any treatment: the trust of his patient. Given greater contact with modern medicine, the traditional physician would be able to bring the best of both medical worlds to the bedside.

Even the Chinese were somewhat startled, I suspect, to find this shotgun marriage of two systems resulting in extraordinary innovations. The first and, as I write, the most striking example, is acupuncture anesthesia. Almost as soon as we arrived in Canton, we were invited to see an operation performed with acupuncture used as the sole means of obliterating pain. It was, for us, an incredible sight, and the surgeon who performed the operation—removal of the lobe of the left lung—later told us that he had not believed in the technique himself. Only after he had seen it used many times on the young and old, the vigorous and the desperately ill, did he acknowledge that traditional Chinese medicine had brought to modern surgery a gift of great price, for acupuncture anesthesia spares the patient many, if not all, of the unpleasant and sometimes hazardous side effects of conventional inhalation anesthesia.

The scene was an operating room that would be familiar to any surgeon. On the operating table was a man of about forty. He happened to be a surgeon himself. Chronically ill with tuberculosis, he had agreed with his colleagues that the only way to cure, or at least to completely arrest, his disease was to remove the diseased lobe of his lung. He greeted us amiably through our interpreter and lay back on the table while the nurses covered him with sterile operating room drapes.

While these preparations were being made, the acupuncturist began. First, she swabbed the patient's right forearm with alcohol and then from a variety of flexible stainless steel needles chose one, which she inserted to a depth of about 2 centimeters into the outer surface of the forearm, about midway between the wrist and elbow. (Watching the patient, I could see no sign that this hurt him at all, and later, when I asked an acupuncturist to use his technique on me, I felt no pain whatever.) The acupuncturist then began a deft but complicated twirling manipulation of the needle, while the patient and his colleagues continued to chat every bit as unconcernedly as if they were discussing some not very important matter. It was almost impossible to believe what was happening. Were these people really going to perform a major operation under these conditions? Would the surgeon-patient really submit to having his chest opened and a part of his lung removed? Surely, I thought, they would take *some* other measures for the relief of pain before proceeding to the incision. But all that happened was that occasionally the acupuncturist or the stand-by Western-style anesthesiologist would interrupt the conversation between the surgeon-patient and the operating surgeon to ask the patient questions about his sensations. Later, I learned that this was how the acupuncturist determines whether the desired feeling of heaviness and a tingling sensation at the site of the puncture were present, since these indicate that the manipulation of the needle is having the correct effect.

About twenty minutes passed before the acupuncturist indicated, by a slight nod to the surgeon, that he could now proceed. I braced myself for the screams of the patient that would surely follow when the incision was made. What happened, however, was something I could never have credited had I not seen it myself, and perhaps not even then if I had not been in the company of two distinguished, level-headed fellow physicians from America.

Without the least hesitation, the surgeon swiftly cut an incision from close to the patient's spine across the left chest wall under the ribs to the breastbone. Then he took a scissorslike instrument with which he cut each rib away from the sternum. With a rib spreader, he separated the ribs from the breastbone, exposing the chest cavity and revealing the beating heart and collapsed lung.

Not a sound. The acupuncturist continued imperturbably twirling the needle with her thumb, forefinger, and middle finger. The patient lay impassively under the knife. Equally calmly, the stand-by anesthetist periodically checked the patient's blood pressure, verified that the patient's pupils were equally dilated, and asked him how he felt. When the incision was complete and the operative field exposed, everyone seemed to pause a moment. The surgeon smiled at the patient, and told him what the situation seemed to be. The next step was to remove the diseased tissue.

Before they went on, a nurse gave the patient a sip of tea from the long, thin spout of a kettle. Then the operation was resumed. The diseased lobe was gently resected, lifted out of the chest cavity, and shown to the surgeon-patient. A discussion followed between the patient and the surgeon. They were considering, the translator told us, whether this was sufficient. Would it be better to take out the whole lung, perhaps? The joint decision was evidently made in favor of the conservative approach, for the wound was closed without further lung resection. Then the patient, fully conscious, smiling, and waving his little red book of *Quotations from Mao Tse-tung,* was wheeled away on a stretcher, but not before he sat up and said goodbye to "the American friends."

It was easy to understand how difficult it must have been for the Chinese surgeons to accept the idea that such a thing was possible. Thinking about it later, I wondered whether the doctors who witnessed the first use of ether in an operation had not been just as dumbfounded by what they saw. That operation, which took place in the operating amphitheatre of the Massachusetts General Hospital in Boston on October 16, 1846, was witnessed by Washington Ayer, who later described the scene this way:

> The day arrived; the time appointed was noted on the dial, when the patient was led into the operating room, and Dr. Warren and a board of the most eminent surgeons in the State were gathered around the sufferer. All is ready—the stillness oppressive. It had been announced "that a test of some preparation was to be made for which the *astonishing* claim had been made that it would render the person operated upon free from pain." These are the words of Dr. Warren that broke the stillness.
>
> Those present were incredulous, and, as Dr. Morton had not arrived at the time appointed and fifteen minutes had passed, Dr. Warren said, with significant meaning, "I presume he is otherwise engaged." This was followed with a "derisive laugh," and Dr. Warren grasped his knife and was about to proceed with the operation. At that moment Dr. Morton entered a side door, when Dr. Warren turned to him and in a strong voice said, "Well, sir, your patient is ready." In a few minutes he was ready for the surgeon's knife, when Dr. Morton said, "*Your* patient is ready, sir." . . .
>
> The operation was for a congenital tumor on the left side of the neck, extending along the jaw to the maxillary gland and into the mouth, embracing a margin of the tongue. The operation was successful; and when the patient recovered he declared he had suffered no pain. Dr. Warren turned to those present and said, "Gentlemen, this is no humbug." [Emphasis in the original.]

No humbug. Exactly the same words apply to acupuncture *anesthesia.* This technique has been in use only a few years in China and is only now being tried elsewhere in the world. All told, I witnessed fifteen major operations performed under this method of anesthesia. All were obviously successful. I watched the removal of a brain tumor, of thyroid adenomas, of part of the stomach, of the larynx, of the tonsils, and of the teeth. Some patients were in condition to walk into the operating room, submit to the operation, and then walk out again—always holding the "little red book."

Not all of the thousands of operations performed in China with the aid of acupuncture anesthesia are successful, I was told. But about 90 per cent are—an astonishingly high percentage. In the remaining 10 per cent, either the patient proves to be panicky and is given conventional inhalation, local, or spinal anesthesia, or, especially in the case of abdominal surgery, acupuncture is discontinued when the surgeon finds the muscles too rigid to permit him to operate properly. In such cases, conventional anesthesia and pharmacology are called into action to bring about the needed degree of muscular relaxation.

In those cases where the patient simply does not feel able to undergo major surgery while fully conscious, his wishes, I was told, are always respected, and I do not doubt this for two reasons: It would be foolish in the extreme to do otherwise, since a serious crisis might follow in mid-operation. And as important to the Chinese doctors, I believe, is their awareness of the damage that would be done to the remarkably close relationship Chinese physicians and surgeons establish with their patients. The whole operating team visits the patient prior to the scheduled operation. There is much discussion of the whole situation of the sick person in which everyone, including the patient and his nearest relatives, participate. This close rapport was always reflected in the operating room and at the bedside, where there was a warmth and trust that is, unfortunately, all too often absent in Western hospitals.

Perhaps the reason why Chinese doctors are so often able to persuade patients to accept acupuncture anesthesia is because they treat them like peers, like responsible members of society who can be expected to act in their own and in society's interests. And the advantages of acupuncture anesthesia are obvious.

Patients can be operated on without delay, because there is none of the risk inherent in giving inhalation anesthesia to a person whose stomach contains food and liquids which, if vomited, could cause death by being inhaled. Furthermore, the powerful chemicals in anesthetic gas mixtures can cause the patient further stress, and can produce irritation of the lungs, followed by pneumonia. Unlike conventional anesthesia, acupuncture techniques also do not worsen the state of shock that an accident victim or desperately ill patient may be in at the time when surgery is needed. Consequently, Chinese surgeons always elect this technique of anesthesia in the severely debilitated, the very young, or those who are in shock.

From society's point of view, the new technique offers the important advantages of ease of execution and of economy. Expensive, complicated apparatus is not needed. Although carefully trained, the acupuncturist has a relatively straightforward duty to perform and need not, therefore, undergo years of training in medical subjects. And for a country like China, the method is particularly valuable because it can be carried out anywhere, in a modern hospital, in the commune first-aid station, or even in the simplest peasant home in the remotest part of the country.

Some of us wondered whether the analgesic effects of acupuncture anesthesia might not be, at least in part, due to the powerful psychological effects of appeals to pride, to the power of the thoughts of Chairman Mao, to revolutionary duty, and so forth. We asked the chief of anesthesiology at one hospital his opinion of these ideas. He smiled good-naturedly.

"My responsibility here is to decide on the anesthetic technique to be used in a given case," he said. "Today's schedule called for six procedures, three using acupuncture anesthesia, one using caudal block, and two using inhalation anesthesia. We use acupuncture anesthesia in a very large number of cases, in patients as young as two years and in the very old. As a matter of fact, I regard it as especially suitable for the young and the aged, whose reaction, as you doubtless know, to conventional pharmaceutical anesthetics is hazardous.

"Frankly, I doubt very much that the two-year-old child is much influenced by the thoughts of Chairman Mao, at least not directly in the sense that your question implies."

He smiled and then added: "Furthermore, we have been investigating this phenomenon in laboratory animals. Electrophysiological studies show that there is a very definite alteration and even abolition of pain stimuli reaching the brain when acupuncture is correctly employed in cats, rabbits, and even a mule. We really don't feel that Chairman Mao's thoughts can be a factor in such situations."

The practice of acupuncture is a very ancient art, but its use to produce anesthesia goes back only to 1966. That was during the Cultural Revolution, when every norm in Chinese society was re-examined. In medicine this resulted in a great upheaval. Medical schools shut down. Mao Tse-tung's call for amalgamating traditional and modern medicine was taken much more seriously.

When the analgesic effects of acupuncture were observed, experiments began to determine what the minimum number of acupuncture points were that would produce analgesia in various parts of the body. Following an old medical tradition, the experimenters performed their first tests on themselves, transferring the results to experiments on their colleagues, and finally trying the anesthetic procedures on patients. It was soon discovered that only a few acupuncture points were critical to the production of anesthesia in a given location. Indeed, as we have seen, in some cases a single needle inserted at precisely the right place and either manipulated by hand or connected to a source of low-voltage direct current sufficed to give complete anesthesia during chest surgery.

At this writing, there is a great deal of speculation both in

China and abroad concerning the way in which acupuncture produces its analgesic effects. It seems likely, however, that it does so by producing an irritation in one part of the central nervous system sufficiently strong so that weaker stimuli are shunted aside and are not perceived in the brain. Something like this effect was described centuries ago by Hippocrates when he wrote: "Of simultaneous pains in two places, the lesser is obliterated by the greater"—although acupuncture anesthesia produces no real pain.

This is not the place to go into greater detail about acupuncture anesthesia. There are two reasons for this: six weeks is not long enough to permit anyone to acquire really precise information about so important a development in medicine; and this is not, after all, a textbook on anesthesia or surgery.

Before going on to other matters, however, I should like to predict that acupuncture will soon be used for anesthesia in Europe and America. Its advantages are so great that the technique will irresistibly sweep over the cultural barriers that still stand between traditional Chinese medicine and what we like to think of fondly as modern "rational" medicine.

But let the Western doctor beware. If he will just stop to think about it, he knows that there is much in modern medicine that is unexplained and much more that is not necessarily as scientific or rational as he likes to believe. Only a few years ago, tonsillectomies were performed almost routinely on young children. This is no longer true. Antibiotics only partly explain why this fad has vanished. The truth is that removing normal, healthy tonsils was an irrational act based on questionable medical theories.

The reverse is also true, in my judgment, when applied to Chinese traditional medicine. The Chinese leaders were quite right in calling the country's doctors' attention to the probability that this body of knowledge must contain many valuable contributions to therapeutics. Certainly, the development of acupuncture anesthesia, which was the direct result of serious inquiry into traditional medicine in China, suggests powerfully that many more discoveries—or rediscoveries—are in store for medicine as we learn more.

One of these discoveries yet to come may be a new approach to a problem that has baffled otologists since long before that specialty was created. I refer to the treatment of nerve deafness. As the reader of this memoir knows, Western otology can do nothing for the patient who has lost the function of the nerve of hearing, either because of congenital impairment or because of an acquired loss. In China today, doctors of the People's Liberation Army are trying to apply acupuncture techniques to the treatment of children with severe neurosensory hearing loss. I visited schools for the deaf in Canton, Peking, and Shanghai and watched the treatments given to the children. The results reported by the P.L.A. doctors in these schools were encouraging, but there was no opportunity for me to learn the details. It would take several months of testing and study of both patients and audiometry records to determine exactly how effective acupuncture for nerve deafness may actually be.

Everywhere we went in China we were invariably invited to offer criticism of what we had seen.

"We realize we have shortcomings," we heard over and over again. "We would appreciate very much hearing any suggestions or criticisms you might have."

At first, I thought this was a mere ritual and offered no comments, but when we visited the schools for the deaf, I was in my own field and criticisms did indeed occur to me. Finally, at one school I commented that the testing procedures were not very precise and so it was not possible to determine with any confidence the true effects, if any, that acupuncture might be having on cases of nerve deafness. The reaction was friendly, even interested. Could I suggest better methods? Of course I could, but they involved using sophisticated equipment that was just not available. I wished I had left my instruments and head-piece at home and had brought audiometers and other testing equipment instead. The interest of the Chinese seemed so sincere that, before we left, I wrote a letter to the appropriate officials of the Chinese Medical Association. In it I proposed that Helen and I return to China, bringing with us audiometers and other instrumentation to permit setting up a really precise study of acupuncture therapy for neurosensory hearing loss.

Not long after we returned to New York, our friend Huang Hua, who by now had been named as the Permanent Representative of the People's Republic at the United Nations, invited me to a conference at the Chinese U.N. Mission. We sat down around tea, exchanged pleasantries, and then got down to the business at hand. My letter had evoked an immediate response. Helen and I were invited to return to Peking with testing equipment and participate in a joint American-Chinese project to study the use of acupuncture in treating nerve deafness.

We brought five new audiometers back to China with us. One was a special high-frequency device similar to the one we had used in Africa. Custom-made by Vincent Skee, this one was designed for use in a Peking hospital where the effects of cardio-vascular disease on hearing acuity in the high frequencies will be studied. Two of the four conventional audiometers were battery-powered for use in the countryside, and the other two were standard audiometers which we turned over to the staff of No. 3 Peking School for the Deaf.

The school is about twenty minutes from downtown Peking. It was established in 1958 by the People's Liberation Army and has about 250 severely deaf pupils, aged nine to thirteen. Acupuncture treatment of nerve deafness did not begin at the school until 1968, but today the school doctors regularly treat the children by this method.

We had planned to spend about a week teaching our Chinese colleagues how to operate the audiometers, including the method of calibrating each of their earphones with the analyzer we had brought along. The precise calibration of each earphone is essential if one is to get accurate data on the hearing of each child. Once again, our Chinese colleagues exceeded our expectations. Instead of taking a week to learn the operation of the instruments, they caught on so quickly that less than two days were needed to make skilled operators of them.

Even before we arrived, the Chinese had planned carefully for us. There were 111 children who constituted the incoming class admitted during 1972. These were to be the subjects of our collaborative study. Because the plan called for our setting up a closely parallel study in New York, Helen and I undertook different assignments at No. 3 Peking School for the Deaf. Helen tested the 111 children and took a detailed history of each of them. Meanwhile, I spent my time with the P.L.A. doctor who performed acupuncture at the school. He was Dr. Fang Yao-sian, a man of about thirty-one, and an expert in his field. He was not a traditional practitioner of acupuncture but was, rather, a good example of the modern Chinese physician who is widely knowledgeable in both traditional and Western-style medicine. He had an M.D., of course, and was systematic in both record-keeping and in his therapy for each child.

Dr. Fang taught me how to do acupuncture for neuro-sensory hearing loss. It is a complex process. There were twenty-two acupuncture points to be learned and used. The treatment consists of using two, or at most three, of these points at each session. The children are treated with very fine stainless steel needles—the standard instrument now used for acupuncture in China—once a day for ten days. Then there is an interval of ten days without acupuncture, followed by renewed treatment for another ten days, and so on.

Dr. Fang and his associates at the school felt that about half of our 111 patients had shown some improvement in the course of treatment. Improvement was judged by an ingenious method of testing he had adopted because he had no sophisticated audiometry equipment until we arrived. In the playground of the school, he had marked off distances of half a meter, a meter, two meters, four meters, and so forth. (A meter is about equal to a yard.) With the child facing away from the tester, the distance at which he could hear a spoken word was determined at regular intervals of time.

Of course the Chinese were delighted at the prospect of retesting all the children using the new equipment. They not only watched Helen closely but also practiced audiometry on each other and on the other children at the school. To make quite sure that the testing technique was reliable in this new setting, we locked up the test results of all 111 children and tested them all over again. When the two sets of tests were compared, 75 per cent of them were virtually identical. We then concentrated on carefully testing for a third time the remaining 25 per cent. When we had finished, we all agreed to take the best result for any child as the baseline from which we plan to make comparisons after about a year of treatment.

Back in New York, Helen and I are now organizing a parallel study of about 100 profoundly deaf children. They will be matched for severity of hearing loss and for age. Of course they will be tested in exactly the same way as their little Chinese brothers and sisters, and, if my training at the skilled hands of Dr. Fang is as successful as I hope it will prove to be, they will also receive the same acupuncture therapy.

By the time this book is published, the study will be under way in America—the first joint Chinese-American medical research project in a quarter of a century. Who knows what will come of it? There will be intercultural differences that may prove both interesting and troublesome. Chinese children are accustomed to acupuncture. They see it performed on adults and children and accept it as a matter of course. It is not painful.

Helen and I have experienced its effects and can testify to that, but American children may be much more diffident about submitting to the needles, at least at first. Furthermore, Chinese children are highly motivated toward self-improvement for the sake of contributing the maximum to their new society. From the cradle they are taught that they must be of service to the people, and when they enter such a school as No. 3 Peking School for the Deaf, they are told that they now have an opportunity to overcome their handicap and become fully useful members of society. Ultimately, my Chinese colleagues and I hope to publish jointly the complete results of our collaborative study of the treatment of neurosensory loss by acupuncture, but that time is still a long way in the future.

Exciting as these developments are, I was most impressed by what is happening in the general practice of medicine, surgery, and public health in China. This, too, is a comparatively recent development, dating from what the Chinese call the "Great Proletarian Cultural Revolution." During this period, Western-trained physicians, surgeons, and health workers were forced to leave their well-equipped hospitals and laboratories and go to live, teach, and work in the countryside. The government's aim was twofold: to bring medical care directly to the masses of Chinese people, most of whom are peasants and who live on communes in the country; but equally important, to re-educate the urban intellectuals, to make them conscious of the life of the peasant, on whose back-breaking labor the welfare of the nation totally depends. Although this mass migration to the country has subsided to some extent today, it is still required that one-third of the staff of every municipal health facility be out in the countryside at any given time.

Such a requirement would be like sending the staffs of our most splendid voluntary hospitals into the worst slums of our cities. Not only to practice there, but to live and work (or go on welfare!) there for extended periods of time. Since my visit to China, I often wonder what effect such a system would have on the average well-heeled American practitioner.

Certainly, in China the system of rotation into the countryside is succeeding in doing more than bring modern health care to the peasantry. In every hospital where we made rounds, watched surgical procedures, and talked with doctors, nurses, and patients, there was always a session during which we sat around a table in a large conference room, sipping the ubiquitous Chinese green tea. Questions came pouring from both directions. I remember asking one young woman doctor—many more Chinese doctors are women than is the rule in the United States—how her experience in the country had affected her style of practice.

"Before I did this," she said, "my main interest was in the diseases we see here at this hospital. Now I no longer see just the disease. I see the patient. I understand what his life is like and what health means to him, and I have a great desire to restore him to health, which is a very different thing from just wanting to cure his disease."

She was a vigorous young person, trained in a Chinese medical school since the revolution. For others, Western-trained, and accustomed to thinking of themselves as members of an intellectual élite, the experience was far more trying. They had led sedentary lives. They had come to think of themselves as special individuals who bestowed the benefits of their superior knowledge on the lowly peasant. They had never experienced the unbelievable hardships of life in China before the liberation, when a farmer, to obtain treatment for a serious disease, would have to sell all he had and put himself in debt to the landlord for years, perhaps for the rest of his life. To them the prospect of living with the peasants, of laboring in the fields, and of being in the last analysis almost wholly dependent on the goodwill of the peasant leaders of the commune to which they were assigned was a disquieting, perhaps even a fearful prospect.

The reality, as is often the case, turned out to be very different from their fearful fantasies.

"Some of us expected to have a difficult time," a surgeon confided to me, "but when we got to the commune, we were received as honored guests. The peasants with whom we shared food and shelter insisted on offering us the best food, the best bed, the best of everything. It was embarrassing."

Field work did these city people no harm, either. It was hard work, but their bodies grew leaner and harder—and their respect for the peasant grew proportionately. It dawned on them that these people for whom they had previously had a kind of benign contempt were literally feeding the cities, including their own families back in the cities. Gradually, the respect developed into strong ties of friendship between peers. The commune workers welcomed the doctors' suggestions regarding sanitation, personal hygiene, training of local "barefoot doctors" and other health workers to staff local aid stations and hospitals.

"Barefoot doctor" is a term of affection in China. It refers to the young, pioneering health worker, whether he or she works on the commune or in the factory, who has shown a concern for the health and welfare of the people as a whole. Thousands of them have been trained in the vast expanses of the Chinese mainland. Working with revolutionary groups, traditional practitioners, and modern physicians, they have virtually wiped out tuberculosis, venereal disease, smallpox, plague, leprosy, cholera, typhus, and other infections that decimated the Chinese in the years before 1949. Having won a clearcut victory over these pestilences, Chinese medicine has now set out to eliminate schistosomiasis, a parasitic ailment which kills or debilitates millions of the Earth's inhabitants.

Since our visit to China, I have speculated many times on the lessons we might learn from the Chinese medical experience. One cannot transplant things from one culture to another without modification and expect them to flourish, but that does not mean that we could not profit a great deal from what the Chinese have to teach us.

I have no doubt that much of the technical and scientific knowledge the Chinese are gradually mining from their centuries-old traditional medicine will eventually find its way into the armamentarium of physicians and other health workers everywhere in the world. Already one can see that process at work in the study and experimental use of acupuncture anesthesia in the United States. As for the other aspects of traditional Chinese medicine, we would do well not to regard them too condescendingly. After all, it was less than two centuries ago that American physicians bled their patients—sometimes, as in the case of George Washington, to death. They routinely prescribed burned toad for various ailments, solemnly declared that foul air was the cause of malaria (hence the name), and prescribed a diet of carrots for jaundice on the magical principle of similarities—a yellow vegetable to cure a yellowing condition. We would do well to be properly modest about modern medicine, since it too contains its quota of sheer superstitious belief, which, of course, we cannot recognize, since we are believers in those very superstitions. In short, there is so much that we do not know that we would do well to look diligently at every source of knowledge. One of these sources is traditional Chinese medicine, which is based on a pharmacology that, for example, recognized the properties of ephedrine in the second century before Christ.

Three centuries before that, Pien Chu'ueh, a Chinese physician, wrote: "The superior practitioner treats what is not yet sick. The mediocre practitioner treats only what is already sick." Preventive medicine, in other words, is superior to our disease-oriented Western medicine, according to the Chinese, and they have taken it very seriously in their vast and enormously successful public health and hygiene campaigns. In the meantime, they did not neglect their sick, or the very young or very old. In the "bitter past," which is how most Chinese refer to a time as recent as twenty-five years ago, there were, for a nation of some 700 million, only about 15,000 Western-trained and 50,000 traditional physicians. Most of the former and many of the latter were found in the big cities. All of them offered their services only to those who had the price.

In less than a quarter of a century, this ugly picture has literally been swept away by the aroused energies of the Chinese masses. Where there was one shabby hospital for an entire county, there are now hospitals for each commune, capable of handling most obstetrical and surgical situations. The number of physicians trained in both modern and traditional medicine has increased enormously, and, as we have seen, they go into the countryside at regular intervals to teach, to work, and to learn.

Earlier in this book I described the philosophy of my dear friend Henry Wallace. There was one point on which we always differed, although at the time I had little information at my disposal which could enable me to counter his point of view. Henry feared the rise of the "yellow men." In his vision of the future, the white race was seriously threatened by the prospect of the awakening of the Chinese giant, and he knew that that was happening with the Communist revolution in China.

Now that I have seen what has developed in China, I know he was wrong. It is true that the world's most populous nation, endowed with the world's most ancient culture, is awakening from a thousand-year sleep, but it is not a monster that is rising from torpor. When liberation came to China, it came almost without bloodshed. Chiang Kai-shek and his followers were driven off the mainland, but most of his armies stayed behind to join the ranks of the People's Liberation Army. The exploiting classes were liquidated, not by executions but by the elimination of their legal rights to live idly upon their fellow men: landlords could no longer collect rent; land was given to the landless and later assembled into communes which have revolutionized Chinese agriculture; and industry was nationalized.

It sounds simple, but of course it was nothing of the sort. The new China is the product of the consummate political skill of her leaders, especially of Mao Tse-tung. Mao is surely one of the greatest teachers of all time, and the essence of his teaching is profoundly moral. He taught that human nature is dualistic, that man is equally capable of utter selfishness and bestiality toward his fellow man or of great self-sacrifices and capacity for cooperation for the common good. Mao believed that political and economic conditions determine which side of human nature will dominate, and from the feeblest beginnings of the Chinese Communist movement, he set out to demonstrate that the "have-nots" of China had nothing to lose and everything to gain by practicing a selfless, cooperative way of life. The China of today, whose millions are no longer threatened by famine or pestilence, is proof of the power of this fundamental idea.

For me another proof is the impression the Chinese people made on me. They are almost curiously quiet. In the operating room, for instance, there was invariably a complete lack of excitement. There was no tension. You never heard the surgeon raise his voice. The Chinese move quietly. There is a kind of basic tranquillity to the pace of life. No one is in a hurry. Children do not run amok, fall down, fight with other children, as we often see at home. They rarely cry. But although the pace is much slower, although no one seems in a hurry, it is evident that the Chinese as a people are steadily and efficiently getting to where they want to go, because of their capacity for self-discipline and close cooperation with one another to reach a common goal.

In China I felt marvelously relaxed. The atmosphere reminded me of our days in the African bush among the Mabaans.

How quiet and peaceful it was. How slowly and quietly the people walked and talked and went about their affairs, carrying heavy loads of wood, preparing their food. There is something about both the Mabaans and the Chinese that makes them seem beautiful, natural people, in close harmony with nature.

Perhaps what I am trying to describe here is a people in touch with the past *and* the present to a degree that most of the rest of the human race no longer is—although we surely can, and must, attain such contact once again.

# Of Old Men and Wise Men

Purely by coincidence, as I reach this last chapter of this memoir I have also attained three-quarters of a century of living on what we now call "spaceship Earth." Seventy-five years sounds like a very exact measurement. It is, in terms of revolutions of the spaceship in its orbit around the sun, but that's about all. In geological terms, it is less than the twinkling of an eye. Even in the life of mankind as a species, it is no more than a fraction of an instant.

And in human terms, seventy-five years is anything but an exact number. It does not say how old I am at all. A cardiologist will say that I am as old as my arteries. Popular wisdom decrees that I am only as old as I feel. The Chinese would say I am as young as I fight. There is a certain validity in the psychologic concept of age. We all know forty-year-olds who feel and act like tired old men, while by contrast there are always among us octogenarians who are full of vigor and life.

Once again we see that the simplest question is often the

hardest to answer. Asking how old a man is becomes a series of inquiries into the ageing process and into psychological dynamics. How does one measure either with scientific accuracy?

In our studies of presbycusis we were inevitably confronted time and again by this puzzling question. By every physiologic criterion, the Mabaans were far younger than "civilized" city dwellers of the same chronological age. We wanted to find out, if possible, why this was so, and the search for answers has taken us far afield.

One of the remotest of these places is a village high in the Caucasus mountains in the Abkhazian Autonomous Soviet Republic. In the town of Sukhumi and the surrounding rural area there live more than 1,700 persons between the ages of ninety and one hundred twenty-eight. They are the object of careful attention and yearly follow-up by Soviet epidemiologists. Their ages have been carefully checked in church records, by baptismal certificates, by reference to historical events, and by using the ages of children, grandchildren, and great-grandchildren as a basis for estimating the age of the old people.

What intrigued us about the very old Abkhazians was their alertness, their physical condition, and their mental and physical capacities. They were old, but they were very much alive. None of them was "retired," though the very old people worked only a few hours a day in the field or the winery. Except for a Mr. Macti, who at the age of one hundred and two was too busy clearing his land to come in to Duripse, the tiny mountain village where we set up our equipment for testing, the aged residents came to see us on foot or on horseback. Curious about Mr. Macti, we went to him, chatted with him in normal tones, and puffed up a mountain path behind his slight, agile figure so that he could demonstrate on a suitable tree his skill with an ax. He saw nothing remarkable in the fact that at an age greater than a century, he was able to fell a tree with a few strokes. These very old people, so full of life, so vigorous, so devoted to productive work and social participation, are a fertile field for more inquiry into the ageing process.

Western medicine is fond of pointing to the increase in life expectancy that has occurred over the past hundred years in the advanced countries. That is a good thing, but I doubt exceedingly that medicine can take much of the credit. Many great medical discoveries have been made, but much has also happened in society. It was not the pediatricians and the general practitioners who insisted on pasteurization of the milk supply in the American cities of the early 1900's. It was the radical women of that time, who formed milk committees and who hounded and pestered public health officials and medical men until they joined in seeing that babies did not die of "summer complaint" because of contaminated milk. Other political forces brought about the reduction of the work week from twelve hours a day and eighty-four hours a week to the eight-hour day and the forty-hour week. It seems much more likely that this achievement by organized labor has done more to create healthy, well-nourished Americans than all of the miracles of modern medicine put together.

Besides, the span of life has not been lengthened. Today's greater life expectancy is due to the fact that a larger percentage of the population in advanced countries live to my age, instead of dying in the first year of life, or before forty. The span of life, however, remains no greater than it was in Hippocrates' time, with certain exceptions.

When you look at those exceptions, the Abkhazians, the Mabaans, the long-lived residents of the remote Ecuador village of Vilcabamba who have been studied by Dr. Alexander Leaf of Harvard, you begin to realize that these people live longer without benefit of modern scientific medicine. The life expectancy of the newborn Mabaan, or Vilcambaño, is no greater than that of his contemporaries elsewhere in the world. In fact, it is less than that of inhabitants of advanced countries. Yet if he or she survives the perils of the first years of life, he has a far greater chance to live long and age gently. His destiny is not an old age of decrepitude, pain, and uselessness. Instead, he fits easily and naturally into his environment, both natural and social.

"In the long run," says Dr. René Dubos, "man might be more successful biologically and find greater meaning to life if he tried to collaborate with natural forces instead of conquering them. Ideally, he should try to insert himself into the environment in such a manner that his technologies and ways of life relate him more intimately to nature. He might thereby become once more part of nature instead of its uneasy overload."

Dr. Dubos, an American bacteriologist and philosopher of science, is speaking from the point of view of Western science. The "man" he speaks of is the citizen of technologically advanced Europe, Japan, or America. Elsewere in the world—in the remote Sudan, the Caucasus, Ecuador, perhaps in Tibet, and who knows where else?—there are men who live according to Dubos's concept of the biologically successful life. For the most part they have to, because they possess no formidable technology like ours to give them, temporarily, the illusion of mastery over nature.

But is it really necessary to befoul the environment in which we must live by the development of an uncontrolled technological monster? The Chinese, who are only now entering the modern scientific era, may have an answer to this question. Shortly after the 1949 revolution, the pressures to industrialize China grew apace. Some leaders of China were convinced that a modern society could, in fact, survive only if a complex technological basis for it were created as rapidly as possible regardless of the cost to the present generation. Others, of whom Mao Tse-tung was one, said an emphatic *No.* He evidently feared that rapid industrialization would keep China in what Thorstein Veblen once called "the predatory phase" of its economic and social development, the stage in which the dominant feature of social relationships was the exploitation of one man by another. Instead, Mao insisted that China "walk on two legs," that she feed herself, clothe herself, and heal herself of the insect-borne and infectious diseases she had inherited from "the bitter past."

As a consequence, China has begun to industrialize only gradually, but even in this aspect of Chinese life one sees signs of a way of life that is more collaborative, as Dubos puts it, with nature.

Perhaps as a result of their thousands of years of civilization, the Chinese seem almost intuitively aware that man, too, is a part of nature, and as such has inherited characteristics of his own that must be taken into account. His biology cannot be changed; only his relationship to others in the society in which he lives can be, and is being, altered, so as to maximize what Albert Einstein once referred to as his "social drives."

"Man is, at one and the same time, a solitary being and a a social being," Einstein wrote.

> As a solitary being, he attempts to protect his own existence and that of those who are closest to him, to satisfy his personal desires, and to develop his innate abilities. As a social being, he seeks to gain the recognition and affection of his fellow human beings, to share in their pleasures, to comfort them in their sorrows, and to improve their conditions of life. . . .*

Describing "the essence of the crisis of our time," Einstein pointed out that

> the individual has become more conscious than ever of his dependence upon society. But he does not experience this dependence as a positive asset, as an organic tie, as a protective force, but rather as a threat to his natural rights, or even to his

---

* *Ideas and Opinions* (New York: Crown, 1954), p. 153.

economic existence. Moreover, his position in society is such that the egotistical drives of his make-up are constantly being accentuated while his social drives, which are by nature weaker, progressively deteriorate. All human beings, whatever their position in society, are suffering from this process of deterioration. Unknowingly prisoners of their own egotism, they feel insecure, lonely and deprived of the naive, simple and unsophisticated enjoyment of life. Man can find meaning in life, short and perilous as it is, only through devoting himself to society.*

Einstein was describing the situation of men living in the capitalist society of today. In the socialist third of the world—including Eastern Europe, the Soviet Union, Cuba, and China—change in the relationship of man to his society is apparent in varying degrees. With all their imperfections, these societies are based upon the part of human nature that is social, rather than solitary. They are, after all, socialist societies, the basic aims of which are to share the product of the land and the factory among all members of society.

I am just another doctor, not a politician or a social scientist, but what I have seen suggests strongly to me that while America has much to give the world in technological and scientific achievements, she has just as much to learn about reordering her society in a manner more appropriate to modern necessity as well as to the age-old social imperatives of human nature. It is time we got on with the job.

* Ibid., pp. 155–6.

# A Note About the Author

*Born in Syracuse, New York, in 1897, Samuel Rosen, M.D., is Emeritus Clinical Professor of Otolaryngology at Mount Sinai School of Medicine in New York City. After studying law for one year at Syracuse University, Dr. Rosen turned to medicine and was graduated from Syracuse Medical School in 1921. Thereafter he took his internship and residency training in otology at Mount Sinai Hospital. Appointed to the Mount Sinai staff as an attending physician, Dr. Rosen established a flourishing practice in New York City.*

*In 1957, five years after he perfected a new, much simplified operation for the restoration of hearing in patients suffering from otosclerotic deafness, a defect of the bony wall of the middle ear, Dr. Rosen received the American Medical Association's Hektoen Gold Medal for original work in medicine, and the same year he received the Pietro Caliceti Award from the University of Bologna.*

*A resident of New York City, Dr. Rosen still practices ear surgery and otolaryngology. On trips abroad, he is assisted by his wife, Helen van Dernoot Rosen. The Rosens have a daughter, Judith (Mrs. Albert Ruben), a son, John F. Rosen, M.D., and four grandchildren.*

# A Note on the Type

This book was set on the Linotype in Granjon, a type named in compliment to Robert Granjon, but neither a copy of a classic face nor an entirely original creation. George W. Jones based his designs on the type used by Claude Garamond (1510–61) in his beautiful French books. Granjon more closely resembles Garamond's own type than do any of the various modern types that bear his name.

Robert Granjon began his career as type cutter in 1523. The boldest and most original designer of his time, he was one of the first to practice the trade of type founder apart from that of printer. Between 1557 and 1562 Granjon printed about twenty books in types designed by himself, following, after the fashion, the cursive handwriting of the time. These types, usually known as caractères de civilité, he himself called lettres françaises, as especially appropriate to his own country.

Composed, printed, and bound by The Haddon Craftsmen, Inc., Scranton, Pennsylvania. Typography and binding designed by The Etheredges.